Inspired Parenting

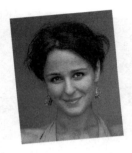

ABOUT THE AUTHOR

Dorka Herner never thought she would use her psychology degree, after she got caught up in the world of media at the beginning of her university years. For two decades she worked as a TV programme editor and a journalist and had her own TV programme and video series. "I was always doing the same thing. I am brave enough to be open and to ask real questions, and as a result, I am aware of feelings, desires, and thoughts being born – in other words, whatever I do, I am a psychologist and a coach."

More recently, Dorka returned to her profession but with a novel approach: "I believe and experience that therapy works best if I don't see it as being only about my clients. Whatever topics they bring to me, I work on those as well. This doesn't mean that I make my concerns visible, but if I don't filter them through myself, I won't notice my blind spots, and I will be a less efficient therapist. My tool is what I call "mirrortherapy": I take the issues raised in a session home with me where I deal with them with the help of sports, breathing exercises, and meditation. By doing this, I am purer and more authentic in the therapist-client relationship. I believe in the strength of acceptance rather than change and I experience how acceptance brings change every day."

Inspired Parenting

*Uplifting insights from a
psychologist & mother of five*

Dorka Herner

Inspired Parenting: Uplifting insights from a psychologist & mother of five

First published 2017 in Hungarian as *Gyerekes gondolatok – Önismereti egypercesek szülőknek* by Jaffa Kiadó És Kereskedelmi Kft

This English edition published by Pinter & Martin Ltd 2020

©2017/2020 Dorka Herner

Translated into English by Nora Toth

ISBN 978-1-78066-485-9

Also available as an ebook

British Library Cataloguing-in-Publication Data
A catalogue record for this book is available from the British Library.

All photographs courtesy of the author.

Set in Adobe Caslon Pro

Printed and bound in Poland by Hussar

This book has been printed on paper that is sourced and harvested from sustainable forests and is FSC accredited.

Pinter & Martin Ltd
6 Effra Parade
London SW2 1PS

pinterandmartin.com

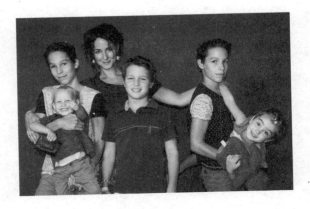

Thank you to Samu, Fülöp, Artúr, Lotti, and Maxim:
the five little people who know me inside out

Contents

Prologue   9

1   Inspired thoughts about everyday situations   11

2   How can I stay well when it's so very hard?   39

3   Reshaping the patterns that shape us   63

4   From the ideal age difference to
    sibling training   89

5   Instead of giving advice on how to raise
    children   113

6   Self-knowledge as a tool   143

    Epilogue   187

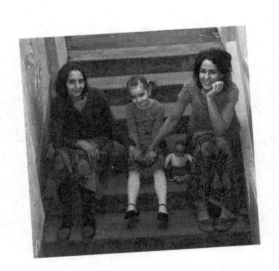

Prologue

I've been a mother of two, then three children. For many years I was a single mother of three; now I'm a mother of five. I have been, and am, a patient mother, an impatient one, one that shouts, and one that asks nicely. I've been a liberal mother and one that's into setting boundaries. I've given birth at home and in hospital. I've been a mother who carried her babies in a scarf and one who pushed a buggy. I've been fat and thin, a brunette and a redhead. I've been single and married. I've had children in state and private nurseries, I've been happy and unhappy. Just like Barbamama, the shape-shifting character in the children's story. At the moment, instead of a blob, I'm more like a peasant woman sitting in the spinning house, sharing moments, thoughts, and stories from my experience as a mother of thirteen years and five children, filtered through a background in psychology and coaching. I don't give advice but that doesn't mean that my book won't be helpful.

1

Inspired thoughts about everyday situations

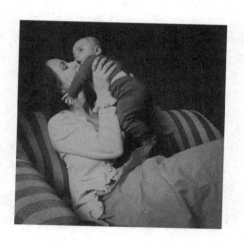

Let's picture a giraffe. Done? When asked to picture a giraffe, eighty-seven out of one hundred people will imagine the same image: a picture of a giraffe's profile. I am one of the thirteen who think of something different. Whether I picture my giraffe in a zoo or in the savannah or wherever depends on many things. It depends on whether I've had a specific experience with a giraffe; on whether I've seen one in its own environment; on whether I've touched one or given it food; on whether I've been bitten or kicked or nuzzled by one. It's possible that as a child, my favourite soft toy was a giraffe and that's what came into my mind. No one flashing picture is better or worse than any other.

Raising children is rather like that giraffe example. Despite there being an infinite number of perspectives, we tend to think about it within a fairly tight framework. This is no accident, and it's not bad either, as looking at things from one perspective makes life considerably simpler. If I don't see all sides of something, but observe only one, I can assess the situation more promptly and with greater ease. If I need to solve a problem quickly, it's important not to weigh up every little thing, as that would take time. But if there's no urgent problem, however, and I have the time, then by seeing it from different perspectives I can access a wider range of options. This then opens up a greater number of choices. I may choose to take the shorter or the longer path; the most enjoyable path or the most relaxing one; the flowery one, the windy one, the wide one, or the one with potholes. They may all lead to the same place, but by taking a different path I change in a different way.

The more experience I have of a certain subject, the closer I get to it; the more I read about it, the more I get to know its dimensions, the more I feel and understand what it is exactly. There is no layer that could not add to my knowledge to some extent. Bringing up children by being physically or mentally abusive is also an option; it's an option many people go for. I see it all the time in the playground, whether it's a smack on the hand or a yell. And it can be effective in making children get used to things or break a habit. Many goals are achievable by it, unquestionably. Still, I wouldn't like to live with this option as I'm aware of the long-term effects. The same way I would not like to put my hand up a giraffe's bum, and I'm not even willing to shake hands with a person who does. Thus, this possible path helps me by indicating which way *not* to go.

My thoughts in writing are like giraffe sketches. I'd like to show you what a giraffe looks like from the top or the bottom. What it feels like to touch. How interesting its eyes are from up close. What it sounds like. How amazingly complex it is on the inside. How it smells. I cannot say which is the best view as there's no such thing. If I get stuck on a single aspect, then I know too little about the whole issue, no matter which aspect I am stuck on. Everything I write down is a possible option, opinion, or thought. And opinions fundamentally different from mine can also be equally valid. What we decide to make use of is up to each and every one of us.

Everyone has an inner structure, a working system, a repertoire of solutions, which can be expanded, shaped, and re-formed. What feels right or comfortable, what can be cut to size, what works for them and their child at the moment, what the value-for-money effect is, can only be judged by the individual. This book offers inspiring thoughts rather than advice. In highlighting different routes, it's basically a tool to make parenting a less bumpy ride.

Good baby?

I'm asked several times every day whether my son is a good baby, a good child. If I don't feel like going into detail, I simply say yes, he is. But I usually take the opportunity to add that in my view all children are good, not just my children. "Does he cry much?" people ask. I usually reply that luckily, he's able to cry. I'd like my child to be well, but not at the price of not crying. If a newborn doesn't cry, that means they're not communicating with us, that they don't expect us to help them feel better, that they don't trust us to do anything for them. A child that doesn't cry feels that they cannot achieve anything. Orphanages are said to be quiet.

And, of course, this doesn't mean that I want my children to cry. Forget that! Who would want to feel like the marrow is being scraped off their spine with a knife? My child crying tears me apart. It drives me mad. I fall to pieces. But that's what they're supposed to do. I don't get salami at the shop if I don't ask for it loud and clear, but simply smile at the shop assistant like a really good child.

Good illness

What I like about snot and coughs is that they don't tie you to one place. You can still go out, see the world, do things. They are sleep-killers though. Diarrhoea is my friend in the short term, but after a while the sight of my kids looking as skinny as cotton buds makes my heart sink. I cope least well in the half-recovered half-sick phase, as I can't keep them busy; they don't have any strength and can be painfully bored. The good thing about fever is that if it's not dangerously high, they cuddle up, slow down, and go to sleep on my lap sniffling. With the bigger children, this experience comes only with fever, so when it does happen, I enjoy every moment of it.

We shouldn't fight in front of the kids?

We shouldn't fight in front of the kids? But we should. If we don't fight and then make up, our children won't have a model of how these things are done. They won't have adequate tools to use in the future. It'll be a frightening, unknown taboo for them. Where can they possibly learn about such things safely, if not from us, their parents? Which fairytale tells them about fighting and then making up, in detail? I may consider it better for my children not to hear raised voices, but they will most definitely detect suppressed tension and sense the volcano that's about to erupt. If I never argue in front of them, though my aim may be noble in trying not to burden them with what is not their load, I actually put far more weight on them. When the basis of a fight is love and not hatred, and if this is not a permanent war but an occasional argument (and I'm not talking about verbal or physical and systematic abuse here!), then they'll be less traumatised by it than they would be if I were to make them see a natural, common occurrence as a sin or something to be ashamed of. Don't fight behind their backs, or after they've gone to bed and you think that they can't hear you. Argue and make up in front of your children so they can see you making an effort and hugging their father or mother and/ or saying you're sorry. Let them see that even though there's tension, there's also love. If they can't see them both present at the same time, they may believe that anger is bad and means you don't love each other.

It's good to fight

There are many techniques to prevent or stop kids fighting and stop parents arguing. There's lots of useful advice, many practical solutions: be proactive, don't judge, divert their attention, let them negotiate themselves out of situations in a systematic and orderly manner. But why are there so many fights in the first place? There must be something good in them. They must have a function. They happen so often, in so many areas of life. It's easier to accept our behaviour, our coping mechanisms, if we can see their uses as well as their drawbacks.

In an argument, I can redefine myself, what I think about a situation, and why I think it. I can set where my boundaries lie and how far I'm willing to go if there are no limits.

When there are no potatoes in the house and I want to make mashed potatoes, when gravity proves too strong and things drop out from my hands, when I'd hoped to spend most of the day at the playground but it's pouring down, when the carpenter is late and it's getting near sleep time... these little "I didn't plan for this" things create tension in me even when I don't feel it, even if I solve the situation brilliantly the first time. And no matter how huge my tolerance pot is, it fills drop by drop, like a bladder, with all the soluble waste that I cannot absorb. And an argument, like the act of urinating, empties me, cleans me out.

We don't find these acts very attractive, and we don't like doing them in front of others. Yet both are extremely useful:

fighting and urinating let us get rid of stuff that stresses us – sometimes for hours, days, even years – in a very short time. This can bring a great sense of relief, a good sort of emptiness. Shouting not only cleans us out, but also clears our relationships: things that have been present in some form of energy for a while and have influenced us invisibly are finally voiced. And it's much easier to create real closeness in a clearer relationship. It's no accident that good sex often happens after an argument. Urine can only leave our body in one way; luckily, tension is not like that. We can empty the pot by playing sports, competitive board games and video games; by wrestling on the floor; or by watching exciting movies. However, it's simpler for me to use members of my family.

The person I fight with, I also feel safe with to some extent. Either because we're in a close relationship or the contrary. If I swear at the taxi driver who nearly hit my car, I'm not afraid that our relationship will suffer. I've nothing to lose. There's nothing at stake. But no matter how angry my boss makes me, it's not safe for me to shout at them as they can sack me. In that situation, I'm inhibited by my existential worries. When my older brother mocks me, I kick my younger brother: it'd be silly for me to have a go at the stronger one as his comeback may be too much to take.

If I choose to fight, I avoid suppressing my feelings, even if suppressing my feelings seems far more amicable. If I can control the tensions hidden within me as if they don't even exist, if I don't free myself of them but suppress them, then they can erupt like a volcano, unexpectedly, with the lava pouring over, burying, destroying everything in its wake.

Arguing shows good things about me. For example, it shows that I'm able to make peace, that I can say sorry, or even if not in the heat of the moment, that I'm able to accept that the other person is right.

I may hate and label a blood-sucking mosquito as bad and useless, but in the wider context I can see that for the frog and the stork to survive, the mosquito is also necessary.

Magnetizing

My son was five years old when, at his grandmother's, he stole things from guests staying at her house. It became known a few days later when he brought me a ten-thousand-forint note as a contribution to a toy he wanted me to buy for him. I asked him where the money had come from. He said it was from his father. I said I found that strange. So, he corrected himself in a transparent sort of way and said that it was from his grandmother. I asked him to tell me the truth. He pulled out a mobile phone, a bankcard, and an ID card from underneath his bed. I couldn't breathe. I asked haltingly what these things were and where they'd come from and anyway, whaaaat?! He told me that when nobody was in the room he took them out of the bags that had been left there. But why, I asked, and why these things in particular? "Because I really wanted some of these adult things." From then on, I let my children play with my mobile, and unload and reload the contents of my wallet. If they can experience these things, if they're not unattainable desires, then they're not magnets that can keep them hooked for months or even decades.

I've also experienced this myself. My brother always mocked me when I was playing with my dolls. He picked on me day and night. I didn't have many dolls or clothes for them. I never got a Barbie because my parents didn't approve of her – it's not my favourite doll now either, but back then I really wanted one. When I was eighteen, my friends gave me a Barbie doll, which my little sister lost the following day at playgroup... It's a pretty rough life for a girl, isn't it? But I've more or less found the solution to living with my desire: I've had five babies of my own. That simple.

Unbearable crying

My baby crying while I'm driving hits one of my most vulnerable spots. I often end up crying myself by the time we get from A to B. It doesn't bother my husband, partly because he's happy in the knowledge that it's unsafe to take the baby out of his seat while we're driving and partly because he is helped by the thought that he'll comfort the baby as soon as we arrive wherever we're going. He's more bothered when the baby cries in his arms and won't stop. I, on the other hand, feel that if I do everything within my power to try to soothe the baby, then his crying doesn't tear me apart. For me, it's the intention that's important here, that my baby can feel that I'm doing things for him, and with my good intentions I feel I already give him a lot. If I manage to figure out what it is that will make him feel better, what will soothe him, that's the cherry on the cake.

My children are really lucky that their mother and father are bothered by different types of crying; at least one parent will be trying to soothe them in most situations. Because one thing that my husband and I share is that we both do everything possible to put a stop to anything that feels like an electric current running through our brainstems.

No strudel

One winter, my daughter and I were walking round and round a square in the snow just like Winnie-the-Pooh and Piglet. We were all wrapped up, singing a rhyme. "If you don't step together, you can't have strudel for dinner." Suddenly, I realised that I didn't want to instill in my two-year-old's subconscious that she must march together with others, that she must be like everyone else, if she wants to get strudel... and high grades... or a promotion... or the year-end bonus. So, we rewrote the rhyme: "If you don't step together, you'll get kisses for dinner, because kisses are very good, everyone should get them, too."

Sometimes we sing this version, sometimes the original rhyme. The option to choose gives us freedom.

The first X

In my older twin sons' primary school, there was a system in place whereby they drew a smiley for themselves if things went well, or an X if things didn't go the way the teacher expected. The first September came and went, as did October, and November. They'd report daily: Mama, I got a smiley again! I was happy, at first very happy. On the tenth occasion, I was still very happy, but by the end of November, I'd become routinely happy.

The day came when the question about what school had been like was greeted with silence. That heavy, deep, succinct silence... you know the one. With much difficulty, finally, they came out with it: "We got an X." I can't remember what they'd done, only how surprised they were that I was happy to hear the news. "Finally", I said, "not that boring smiley! Finally, some change!" They now feel safe at school; they don't try to behave eight hours a day. Finally, they have the courage to be themselves. Yippee!

Never mind

Never mind. Never mind. I say this to my child who is throwing up, to the one who has fallen over and hurt their knee, to the one who has not been accepted at the school of their choice, to the one who got bad grades, to the one whose favourite cup has broken. But besides comforting them, what message am I actually passing on? I'm telling them that their problem is not so bad and that they shouldn't get upset about it. I'm downgrading their physical/emotional difficulties even though I can't possibly have any idea about the pain they're experiencing. Of course we mind. We mind because they're feeling bad even if we don't consider the situation so grave.

I often soothe myself with a "never mind." Sometimes I get scared with my child and just as my mother used to comfort me with these words, I use them as well. It's important that I am calm so that I can offer my child more security, but perhaps I could achieve this in another way, for example by taking a slow, deep, silent breath.

Whenever I can, I choose various, perhaps clearer calming techniques that don't have any undertones: You poor thing. I'll hold your head or get a plaster. We'll find a solution together. I'll sign off on that bad grade. I understand… I'm here for you. I can also ask questions: Does it really hurt so much? Can I do anything for you?

With these, I can achieve what I'm aiming for with my "never mind" in the first place: understanding, support, and safety. Unfortunately, I can't take away my child's pain and sadness. Even if I could, perhaps I'd decide not to. Because without the falls, they'll not learn to walk alone. And because it's not at all certain that I'd take from them the ones that bother them the most, or the ones that cause the most pain. The intensity of feelings can never be judged accurately from the outside, as nice as it would be to have a trouble-meter next to the thermometer.

Cry and let it all out

There are few credos I consider as harmful as this one: "crying is for babies." Don't show your feelings, you fool! Suppress them. Let the tension split you in two. But don't show how you feel, not under any circumstances. Grin and bear it. Don't cry! It's a man thing, so act like a man, especially if you're a boy. Girls may be forgiven for fussing, but a boy, no matter how young he is, must really try to be a man!

I don't tell my children not to cry when more than one drop of blood per minute leaves their body. I consider crying justified then. But is it always the most severe injury that bleeds the most? Our tongue bleeds much more than the rest of our body, but hitting our shinbone can still hurt a lot more than biting our tongue.

Emotional pain is a thousand times more complex. It's not easy to listen to crying, but it's good to cry because it's useful, because tears clear away pain, tension, anger, and sadness. Crying and showing emotion are not only allowed in our house, but also highly recommended.

Nursery school signs

With my first two children, I believed that the signs they were allocated at nursery school would have a considerable effect on their lives.* They wanted a hockey helmet and a hockey stick, and I was terribly disappointed that they were fobbed off with a bear and a cat. With my third, having his wish fulfilled and getting a guitar felt fantastic. Yeah, we got it right the third time! With my fourth, I was unable to attend the parents' evening when the signs for each child were chosen, and I was worried what would happen if she were left with that lame little mushroom – which was also my nursery sign. There'd go her future. I asked her what sign she would like to get. "I don't care what it is as long as it's drawn in purple." After all these years of studying psychology and doing tons of work on myself, I was still learning from my child who was not yet three: everything can be turned around in a way that suits us just fine.

"It doesn't matter what happens to you, the main thing is what you do with it." I heard this from Robi Damelin, an Israeli mother whose twenty-eight-year-old son was shot by a Palestinian man, after which she became an advocate for Israeli-Palestinian peace. She explained that the only road to processing the trauma, to gaining acceptance and inner freedom, was to not stay a victim by getting stuck in anger. These words carried enormous weight, especially after what she'd been through. They captured me. They stayed with me. I use them when I get

---

* In Hungary, all children entering nursery school are allocated an image of a common object, their "sign". As they cannot read, this image is used to mark their personal objects throughout the three or more years they spend at nursery (between the ages of 3 and 6). These signs are typically toys that children play with, such as a spade, a bucket, a teddy bear, a doll, everyday objects such as a chair, a table, a book, or plants and fruit such as a pine tree, a mushroom, an apple, a bunch of grapes, etc.

a tiny bit stuck or when I'm faced with great difficulties. I recall the words, looking at my own problem through the sieve of her sentence. These words help me find ways to deal with situations, ways I don't think about when I'm angry, tense, or when I'm stuck somewhere, even in joy.

For example, the decision to write a book was born at a time when I felt as if I'd been set in concrete up to my chin. I was immobilised by two under-threes and three schoolchildren with their daily routines, by childhood illnesses that had been going around for weeks, by the hopelessness of our finances. On top of all that, I'd just found out that my twins had been accepted by the private secondary school they wanted to go to, with its crazy fees that we couldn't afford. So, what now? I asked myself. They can't go? This is what they'd been dreaming of, what they'd been fighting for. And I was the one accompanying them on this road, repeatedly telling them to fight for their dreams, to dare to be themselves, that it was okay to make mistakes, that the important thing was that they believed in themselves. And now that they'd achieved their dream, should I say... um, sorry, everything I said is still true, but could you go to a public school with no tuition fees? Would my telling them to fight for their dreams in the future have any credibility? Would they retain their ability to dream and fight if they could not enjoy the fruit of their success today? Could I do it to them and to all their siblings, who were also witnesses to the process and were being shown an example? Could I give up and say that I couldn't find a way to make the money for the fees? I didn't think so.

I knew we'd have to change some aspects of our lives. So, I thought on it. I knew that I could get a job, but I didn't want to put the one-year-old into nursery. I didn't want somebody else to hear his first words. I didn't want to miss the irretrievable jungle of experiences that his first years of intensive development had to offer me if I accompanied him on his journey of discovery in the world. I wanted to hold him after the occasional painful fall as he took his first steps and I wanted to be there clapping my hands when he played football for the first time. This was just as important for me as the dreams of my older children. It was also important for the one-year-old as I believed that the best place for him was with me. I knew, too, that a decision so far removed from my value system and my wishes would drag me down. And if I were dragged down, I'd also take the other members of the family with me, down to the dark, heavy mud. So that was not the way forward for us. But in which direction should we go?

I recalled Robi Damelin's words. As I said them to myself, I looked at how I could shift from this place I was wedged in. How could I come out of it well? What was it that this difficulty was helping me with? There had to be an advantage and a reason for it, but where and what was it? I paced back and forth, two metres each way, like a tiger locked in a cage, with my feverish child tied to my body. I walked back and forth for five minutes, fifteen minutes, an hour. I couldn't find the answer, I couldn't see it. I was looking at it over and over, concentrating with all my strength, determined not to take the easy way out and let the situation bury me.

And then out it popped: I'll write a book! I instantly felt that this was the perfect solution for me and for us. I enjoyed writing. This was the kind of work I could mould around the needs of my family. But what to write about? Gladwell's *Outliers* comes to mind. If I've done something for 10,000 hours, there's a good chance that I could be good at it. I took my phone, found the calculator, and calculated: my oldest sons were twelve so that's twelve × 365 days, × twelve hours a day (there were many night shifts as well, and there was also the pregnancy, but I didn't count those). As a conservative number, I figured I had 52,560 hours of parenting experience. And I'd been a psychologist for much longer than that.

I wasn't going to be a victim of my life even if it was damn hard. It was a question of motivation, of the time and energy invested, and of the perseverance needed to find the possible avenues I could take and then to choose one that could bring the most happiness. If it didn't bring joy, then I'd carry on searching.

Twinrobics

What is good about having two babies of the same age suffering from colic? Well, I can finally achieve within a few weeks what I'd wanted to achieve when I worked out at the gym for many years: muscular arms, and strong, shapely legs.

Changing perspective

Sometimes I go down on all fours into a frog pose to see what my son, who is only just crawling, can see. It's really rough! Tables are so far up. Giants talk to me from on high. It's an unbelievably long way from one room to the other on my knees. After experiencing this change in perspective, sometimes I remember for weeks to squat or pick him up when I'm talking to him. Or I go to him when he's crying three metres away instead of telling him to come to me.

I experience my oldest kids' perspective through time travel. I recall my adolescent memories about how I was locked into my own perspective by my hormones. Many times, when I didn't say hello to the neighbours, they thought it was out of ignorance while I'd simply failed to notice them. When I walk into to my adolescents' room and say something, it's as if they haven't heard a thing. And that's because they haven't. So sometimes I choose to chat with them online from the adjacent room.

Adolescence

Now and again, living with an adolescent is like having a virus that causes vomiting and diarrhea – the one experiencing the symptoms finds it shitty, but it's not much fun for the person holding their head, either. The repulsive stuff pours out of them at unpredictable times in unpredictable places and then it must all be cleaned up. There's nothing that will help them get better. There's no remedy, except time. We just have to grin and bear it and it'll pass.

Nobody will make you happy

No one can make me happy, and I won't be able to make my children happy, either. How rough is that?! I thought that I could give them happiness. I thought that other people could give me happiness. I spent years walking around in this swamp. Why didn't I deserve to be made happy by somebody? Why couldn't I be the most superb mother, capable of securing the greatest happiness for my family?

After the birth of my fourth child, it finally dawned on me. I realised that no one making me happy could be something completely wonderful instead of being traumatic because it meant that only I could make me happy! And by not being dependent on an outsider for my happiness, I was omnipotent in my own life, limited not by the starry sky, but by my inner confines. As soon as I saw this, I could step out of the victim role, leaving behind the bog of my repetitive actions, stepping out of the unchanging. I took my fate into my own hands and was glad that I'd never need anybody to make me happy. And I realised that the key to my children's happiness was also in their own hands. As a parent, my job is to trim their branches (their dreams) and their buds (their attempts) as little as possible and to let them grow (without creating unnecessary inner limits, fears, anxiety), to make sure they get plenty of light (let them see and experience how enormous and colourful the world is), plant them in rich soil (unconditional love), and give them water (or tea or hot chocolate).

Standby

Detecting the traces of yet another night shift on my face, many ask why I don't have a nap in the afternoon when the kids are also asleep. It's not only because adult time is such a treasure that I find it hard to deprive myself of it. Nor is it the fact that there is no "off" button on the children, so during their afternoon sleep I'm still on call, as they may wake up at any moment. If I expect them to be sleeping for an hour and a half to two hours and I relax a little, if I let myself fall asleep and am woken up after half an hour, I feel irritated. And then the rest of the day is tainted by this irritation or the disappointment I feel. I have to put all my energy into pulling myself together and making it back to point zero. The chance of an afternoon sleep might seem all glitter and gold, but in terms of value for money, it falls far from being a good deal for me, unless I'm really beat.

Looking forward to my retirement

There are times when I'm unable to enjoy the present. It's so difficult that I long for all my children to move out. In our case, that's about twenty years from now. I'm looking forward to my retirement. I'm looking forward to not having to put anyone to bed. I'm looking forward to not having to breastfeed, to change nappies. I'm looking forward to not being pulled apart by any more boundary-testing episodes. I'm looking forward to going on holiday with my husband, even if only for three days. I imagine myself sitting on a sunny Cuban beach with my feet being washed by the turquoise sea. I'm digging in the warm sand. Closing my eyes, I give myself over to the moment while I'm talking to my husband about how lovely it was when we used to put the little ones and the even smaller ones to bed. When they rested on us, panting. I reminisce about how great it was when all five of them sat at the table a couple of times a day and hoovered up large quantities of food in seven minutes. Or when they cuddled up to me during story time. It's a very useful game, time-travelling with my desires; it shows exactly what it is that's so great in the here and now.

Playground

For many long years I used to frequent a playground twice a day. I've had plenty of opportunity to hear the words and sentences uttered by parents, words that are very far from my world. When my three oldest children finally grew out of the playground, I felt that there was no God who could make me set foot in a playground again.

Then I had the two little ones. They love the playground, of course, so I gave in. Maybe not twice a day, but a few times a week, I pop up near the slides. I bury the children's feet in the sand again. I carry water for the pebbles. And I listen.

"I'll leave you here if you don't come."

"Next time, I'll hit you just as hard as you hit your brother."

"If you throw the sand one more time, I'll throw it in your eyes and then you'll see...!"

"See how nicely other children are playing while you're just playing up here?!"

"Santa is not going to bring you anything if you come down that slide again!"

I never share my thoughts or opinions. Everyone messes up their child the way they choose to. However, for me not to be consumed by these sentences, which I find hurtful, I must convert the situation and see it as something different from what it is. So, I sit on the side of the sandpit with a smile in the corners of my mouth, thanking God or whoever that I didn't have parents like that.

Invisibility

One of the best working tools I have with my children is when I'm transparent to them, when I show my feelings, when I communicate openly with them. However, as I don't believe in extremes, I'm also interested in what I can use when I choose to do the exact opposite. Can invisibility also be good?

Sometimes transparency is so scary or shameful, even so

painful for me that I don't have the courage to st(
invisible. For example, if I, or someone important to me, ..
seriously ill, I become upset, tense, and jumpy. I start feeling
frightened and anxious. I'm unable to tell the kids the bad
news. I simply can't find the words. I may choose to pretend
that nothing has happened, but knowing myself, I realise
I'm not really good at this – I can't suppress my feelings
effectively in the long term. I also know that at some point
they/I will erupt. So, I decide on a halfway option. I tell the
children that I'm not too well, but it's not because of them
and for the time being I don't want to say more about it.
They're reassured that whatever it is, it's not to do with them
and so they don't feel anxious because of it. And I wait for
the time when I have the words, when I can find a little
island within me that I can stand on to take courage in order
to show more of me and share the facts.

When my mother* was taken by the police in the autumn
of 2010, we didn't know what would happen, only that it was a
serious matter. We were unable to talk to her. No one gave us any
solid information. There was only a chilling fear. I didn't tell the
children immediately. Until I knew whether she would be kept
in, I didn't want to explain the situation to my two six-year-olds
and my four-year-old. I didn't have the words. All there was,
was a scary dark fog inside and out. When we found out that
she would be kept in prison, it was obvious that I would have
to tell the children that very day. But I didn't know how. I was
sitting on the carpet watching them play with their plastic
toys thinking about how to do this in child language. How
would I begin? What would I do and how would I do it?

Without knowing him, I called the Hungarian child

---

* My mother is Dr Agnes Geréb, gynecologist-obstetrician, independent
midwife, psychologist: www.otthonszules.hu/agnes-gereb

31

psychologist Jenő Ranschburg, and asked for his advice. He told me not to lie to them. Lying to them had never occurred to me for a moment, but which words should I use? Simple ones, he advised. Say that there are good and bad people. Their grandmother is a good person who is being hurt by bad people and this also hurts us. I didn't need to outline this very complex situation to children of this age in detail. He also suggested that I should tell them that it wouldn't be for long. But I couldn't say this to them as I wasn't certain it was true. My advisor agreed I was right and suggested I explain to them how much this was hurting me, too. It was very important that they saw my feelings, if not the facts, in all their complexity.

I don't always want to make the good visible either. For example, when I found out that I was expecting another child, I didn't tell the children immediately. For a few days or weeks, I enjoyed holding on to this secret with the love of my life, planning, being happy, exchanging smiles, not answering questions, just the two of us levitating again and again. I was waiting for a suitable occasion, the right time in me that I could share my joy. I feel similarly about surprises. I enjoy keeping it a secret that I'm planning a holiday because I love seeing the happiness on everyone's faces when I make the announcement. Rather than say "I'm planning a holiday for all of us", it's far better to say: "We're going on a seaside holiday in five days."

Characteristics

If I describe my child as determined and driven, then I can see the good in what I label as stubborn at other times. Brave or hasty, a gourmet or a fusspot: positive and negative sides of the same thing. But the way I label a personality trait indicates my judgement rather than qualifies the people themselves.

Lazy. What a judgemental expression that is, but what does it actually mean? That they are not doing something all the time? If I say this about someone, what I'm really saying is that they are useless. Even though it is so good not to do anything sometimes. I'd like a lazy child. Yes, I'm able to appreciate that even when they are not doing what I want them to, I can simultaneously see and feel the aspect of relaxation and how much this can take them forward.

I make judgements by labeling, whether the label is negative or positive. That's why it's hard to deal with judgements: they reflect the value system of those who use them, yet they're attached as if I were responsible for them. I always felt embarrassed when people said I was beautiful. After a while I learnt to say thank you, but for a long time as a diversion I used to just say that my looks were down to my mother and my father only.

Of course, this does not mean that I never tell my children that they're beautiful, clever, or untidy, I just change the proportion and I say more often that I'm proud of them or that when I look into their eyes I am flooded with warmth or when I look at their desks I'm flooded with anger.

I give by not giving

He fancies the long-life bread, but after the second slice I convince him to have the fresh bread instead, explaining that the latter has less stuff in it that's harmful to our health. He gets it. He switches over. He takes my advice. But to notice in the moment that I do the right thing in the long run by not giving him what he asks for there and then is not always that simple – the closer it is to the soul, the harder it is for me. Naturally, he's on the defensive using his own weapons. I can handle reason and logic easily, but when he puts his sad puppy eyes into action, I have to really try to stay strong. It helps to recall an event when my desires were not fulfilled and in retrospect I can see the advantages of that.

A few years ago, we found ourselves in a very difficult position, financially as well as spiritually. I visited my father for some support and understanding, and as I shared all the details with him, I got angrier by the minute. I expected him to join me in my cursing, and just like me, to get angry with the person responsible for all this. I'd imagined he'd commiserate with me, give me some sympathy. I'd been certain I'd get all these. I had all the aces. But what did he do?! He didn't feel sorry for me. He didn't go crazy with me. He didn't snarl at anyone. Instead, he said in a calm voice: "That's rather unpleasant, indeed, but it's not tragic; tragedy is sickness and death." What??? To all this horror, that's the reaction I get?! I thought I didn't hear him right, and a whole flow of complaints got stuck in me. At first, I was angry, as the situation didn't go according to plan and that was extremely frustrating. I needed a few hours to notice what I'd been given by my father: crutches I've been using ever since. He didn't help me in the moment; he didn't serve my short-term needs; instead, he gave me something that has become my foundation stone. When it's hard to accept a situation or to move on, there's no occasion on which I couldn't make use of his words to give myself a kick in the butt, just enough to move me beyond the deadlock I find myself in.

It's good to have a little me time

The tasks I'm not willing to hand over to anyone fill my days like an amoeba. There's little attention and time left for me. How can this be good? Well, it makes me prioritise. It makes me see the things that are really important to me. Let's say, for instance, that I love being alone. I have two free hours but spending time with a friend is also an option – undisturbed conversation is high on my list of desires. First, I don't decide instantly, leaving myself time to consider, or rather feel in my stomach, which one I long for more. Even when I have the time, I rarely see anyone whose company takes more than it can give. I weigh up many small factors and prioritise the level of emotions. Having time does not necessarily mean that I'm available.

Generally speaking, it appears that the more children I have – and the more my time is filled with motherly duties – the easier I find it to say no, the less I'm looking to please. The little amount of free time available has made me hungry for myself: I've become highly motivated to move towards my own desires.

Predictability = security

I'm unable to give unlimited patience to my children and when I lose my temper, I sometimes shout at them. For a long time, I saw this as one of my major flaws. It's true that I usually warn them in advance and say that I only have the patience to ask nicely two more times and then I'll shout but I don't see those as extenuating circumstances. When I got home one day my son pushed his head into my belly, sobbing.

"What's the matter?" I asked in surprise.

"Papa shouted at me!"

"Oh, my sweetheart, are you really so upset about papa shouting at you? But I shout at you a thousand times and you don't usually get so distressed!"

"That's true but you always tell me that you'll ask nicely two more times and then you'll shout when I really do something wrong. Papa shouted at me when I didn't do anything wrong and he didn't even warn me in advance!"

If I know what to expect, that gives me great security, even when it comes to being shouted at.

Double bond

When my youngest son was born, my husband didn't have much work and this situation would remain unchanged for the next eighteen months. We're a big family, with expenses that go with that. Luckily, the kids are growing. Luckily, there's no problem with their appetite. Luckily, they're extra-open to the world – and for us to be able to meet their needs day by day, maternity pay is not sufficient. From this starting point, I could have chosen to spend the newborn days and months of my youngest child's life worrying about our subsistence. I could have stressed about what was going to happen when our reserves ran out, what would happen if I couldn't borrow from my family and my friends. Still, most of the time I didn't worry. Partly because I'd grown up in a supportive family, which has given me a background and a safety net so at the bottom of my heart I hold a certain feeling of security, even if I worry sometimes. It's inconceivable that we'd end up on the street or not have food on the table.

I can see in those minutes, days, months, years, what it is I had to be thankful for in that transitory period of unemployment: my son got to bond early, not just with me but with his father, too. Apart from breastfeeding, we shared all the tasks. He slept for an hour and a half to two hours on his father at least once, but mostly twice a day. Two people provided security for him. When he smiled, two pairs of eyes took turns to smile back at him. When he cried, two people were there to comfort him. This did not mean that we were both constantly there for him twenty-four hours a day, but rather that we took turns, so that most of the time our child got the person who had the most energy, who could do better at the time.

We could have had a better car or travelled more often, I wouldn't have minded either. But we still had time for those things. This, however, was only possible at the beginning; early bonding has a finite timeframe. It cannot be repeated ever again. It cannot be made up for, emotionally speaking. No such foundations can be laid with the child years later. Nor can such a connection be forged between parent and child.

Our son is as round as the sun and shines just as much. He's no better than the others. He isn't any cleverer or more curious about the world. He simply beams from having rock-solid foundations. He is nowhere near being able to sit up on his own yet he's already standing on both feet.

What to say instead

Are you deaf? It doesn't feel good that I've already asked you several times.

If you cry like that, I'll start crying as well! I feel helpless when I cannot comfort you.

You should be ashamed! I'm very angry and disappointed.

The world doesn't revolve around you! I'd like you to learn to pay attention to other people's needs, too.

Say sorry! It's really painful for him when you hurt him. If you're angry, you can hit the pillow instead.

Don't be so stupid! I don't understand why you've done that. I'd like you never to do it again.

Are you mad?! Gosh, I was so scared! Please don't do this again because it can cause big problems. This is not allowed, I've told you many times before.

Eat it or I'll stuff it down your throat! I'm angry that you're pushing the peas from side to side on your plate and I'm worried that you don't eat enough healthy food.

As long as you live under my roof... You've overstepped the mark so I'm feeling powerless and frustrated, but I'd like us to be able to change this.

2

How can I stay well when it's so very hard?

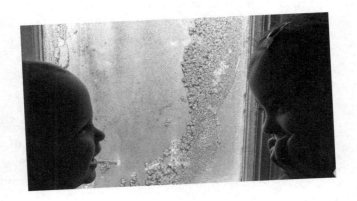

Being with children is like a marble slab: beautifully exciting, valuable, varied, and really hard. Is there a parent out there who has never felt such overwhelming powerlessness and hopelessness that they would happily exit parenting through the nearest window? Is there a woman on the planet who hasn't asked herself within six months of giving birth whether she'd been mad to have longed for this? How can something be so enjoyable, so beautiful, and so joyful and yet so trying? How can parents not get overwhelmed by negative emotions?

Is there a parent in the world who doesn't experience one of the following feelings at least once a week?

- Guilt about not being able to do well enough
- Guilt about not being good enough
- Being overwhelmed by tasks
- Being torn apart by trying to give everyone and everything enough attention (either in relation to siblings or family and work commitments)
- The need to live up to personal or social expectations
- The need to live up to their own expectations

I experience all of them daily, even if just for a short time. I still hurt myself with each one of them. I have no doubt that there's no job harder than being with a child, twenty-four hours a day, seven days a week – and to be well at the same time, too.

Workplace

Mine is the kind of workplace where the boss decides what time I should wake up – as well as sharing my bed. I'm in service instantly. While opening my eyes, I'm making tea as ordered… in my nightie. While having a shower, I'm putting on a puppet show from behind the curtain, throwing bath toys on the floor in front of the boss in the hope of winning a few more minutes for myself. Sometimes I have a poo with the boss sitting on my lap. I make animal sounds on sunny and overcast days. When he's resting, I guard his peace. There are no ten-minute breaks or lunchtimes. Sometimes it feels like being on overtime from first thing in the morning. I'm also on night duty, as the boss may decide to call and check on me at any time either by asking to be fed or by coughing or by having a nightmare. He never lets me switch off completely. The advantage of constantly being on standby is… well… I can't think of one. There's daily pay: a smile, a sentence, a hug, or a cry – being given tears is a big thing. But the time and energy I invest often brings returns only ten or fifteen years later. And there are months – the terrible twos and adolescence – when I'm the one paying the price. So why is this whole parent thing so bloody marvellous?

Everybody knows best

Grandmother, sister, friend, health visitor, my own mother, other people's mothers, everyone knows best. One book says this, another says the exact opposite. Let's say I get stuck with colic. Some suggest I tie the child to me and feed them a lot. Some say the feeds should be at least three hours apart, as colic is caused by air swallowed when breastfeeding. A third source recommends some magical liquid while more swear by the winding pipe (a gas and colic reliever) – I swear it exists. A few weeks later, I'm living on toast, as some forum commenters found this helpful.

One day I'm doing this, the next day I'm doing that. The only thing I'm not doing is listening to me. I'm lost among all the advice. What can I sense my child needs? What is it that helps me get through this phase? Well, these are the voices I can't hear when I'm focusing too much on the outside. It's hard not to be adequate and not to hope that one method or another will actually help. Still, beyond a certain point, bouncing from one idea to the next will probably take me further away from the solution. I'm his mother. I spend the most time with him. I know the most about him, so I'll know best what can help him.

If I manage to listen to my inner voice and find a solution or simple acceptance, the success will be mine alone. And why is this so important? If I try all the advice – if I bathe him in warm water as my grandmother said, if I use the winding instrument recommended by the pharmacy, if I give him the magic drops bought by my friend, if I hold him with his feet up as I read on a website – and finally things improve, then it seems like all those outsiders solved the problem together and I was just the executive instrument. Asking for advice and gathering information is fine. But the decision about which advice to follow should be mine based on my intuition. If I don't do so, I can easily lose my competence – not in front of others but in front of myself. I take the chance of finding my inner security out of my own hands. I must believe that I'm a competent mother to my child. I must find a way to do things, even when it takes longer than three minutes, three weeks, or three months to find a solution. It's worth the struggle, even if it means a little more crying. It's worth it for my child as well, because from then on, he'll be getting more reassurance from me. I must be reborn as a mother; only I can give birth to my own motherhood.

Trauma-wisdom

Have you had a miscarriage? The baby must have been sick, you should be glad you didn't have it! Or: You'll have another one; it's lucky that you're still so young. Have you given birth and it wasn't a good experience? You should be grateful it wasn't a caesarean. Was it a caesarean? You should be glad the baby's alive.

All of these words of intended comfort really are worthless when you've just miscarried or had a traumatic birth. Of course, all these statements can be true – on a cognitive level. However, in a freshly traumatised state, a silent embrace or a gentle stroke or simply saying "I cannot imagine what you've been through and what's going on inside you right now, but I'm here for you and I love you" can help more than any piece of wisdom.

Sleep time

For a long time, I thought that children slept so that I could make lunch, hang out the washing or do the shopping online. It took me years to realise that their sleep time could be measured in gold and is in fact a breath of opportunity for me to recharge, a tiny little exit point from the noise of their activities, time for my grown-up things: reading, sex, doing nothing, watching a TV series, eating in peace, peeing alone, talking to friends, whatever I feel like doing. If I don't take time for me, I should do it for the kids, so that I have enough energy later to reinvest in them.

My weak point

When I'm counting on the small kids to fall asleep at the same time and it doesn't happen, when I'm counting on her sleeping an hour at least in one go but in twelve minutes she asks for a feed again, when I'm counting on getting home in fifteen minutes but it takes thirty-three due to heavy traffic, when I'm counting on my husband to bring bread home and he forgets, when I'm expecting to wake up well-rested but instead I wake up with a headache – all these things irritate, upset, and anger me terribly. What's my solution? The only one that has worked for me so far is not to count on anything at all. Because when I do, I map out my schedule and my energy so that I'm maxed out. I don't leave anything in reserve. I don't leave any room for maneuvers. If I expect that anything anywhere may change from where I have put it in the plan, if I give things some room to move, I free myself from disappointment. I remain more flexible and my days become more enjoyable.

Surely it would be a good solution if I just gave myself more leeway, but I find that much harder.

I snatch snippets of sleep

I've read that research has proven that only the left hemisphere of the brain actually sleeps for the first night when at a new place because the right one is on guard. I think only the left hemisphere sleeps in mothers of small children as well for the first year(s). I'm on standby at night too, woken by every stir. It takes me five seconds to get from my bed to the child throwing up in the next room, including the time it takes to pick up a bowl from the bathroom on the way.

You can get used to this dolphin sleep, but it takes its toll. The good news is that every day I'm closer to the time when they'll not need me to keep guard. The other good thing is that the hour or two a month when I can definitely sleep undisturbed can work wonders. The regenerative abilities of mothers far exceed those of an Ironman.

Mountain climbing

When he's still enjoying himself at a birthday party, when he's not yet hungry at the playground even though it's nearly lunchtime, when he's still engaged in carefree play but it's way into bath time, when I'm having a great chat with my friend and he's also happy to play – in such situations I find it difficult to make the decision and say "That's it, come on, let's go, we're off." It's hard to move him or myself away from what is so good. But I've learnt that for the day's house of cards not to collapse on me, for him not to be starving on the way home, not to be so tired as to fall asleep in the car, to be able to go off on his own to wash his hands without me dragging him like Christopher Robin does Winnie-the-

Pooh – I must do so. Because as wonderful as it is being on top of the mountain, we still need to come down. And this requires not only time but energy as well, both from me and from my child.

Divorced mother of boys

I'll never enjoy playing football, wrestling, or playing hockey. I'm happy to watch for a while, but I'd rather be a cheerleader. If testosterone were on sale at the shop, I'd buy family-size packages. I'd throw the boys over my shoulder, defeat them with a light sabre, buzz them like a tractor, or fly like a daredevil. I'd be a muscular hero. I know in my mind that it's enough for me just to be their mother, but I still try. If they couldn't spend time with their father, I tried to import testosterone supplements – grandfathers, coaches, uncles, the neighbour's tomcat – and this helped them fill the void. What helped me is when I realised that no matter how hard I tried, I'd never be a man.

Mine is much bigger!

After a difficult morning, we fell through my mother's door in tatters. I could hardly wait to drop off my kids and go out. But where? Anywhere. To breathe. My aunt, sitting in the room, asked what was up.

"Well, I've just got through a really tough evening, a not too easy night, and a truly trying morning," I said, looking for some understanding like "You poor thing. That's how it is. You just have to try and survive." But that's not what I got.

"I can remember that period. I didn't even have a grandmother around to help and I was also working, and on top of all that in my time there were no washing machines!" I sat there scolded, not knowing what to say to this. All I managed was: "Okay, but I've got five kids while you had two." And her counterargument followed, of course: "But your three older ones are big enough, so they're no bother!" "No bother?!" My eyes widened. "Can you remember what it's like living with a teenager?!" And so we carried on until one of the kids sitting on our laps finally spilled something, giving us a reason to stop the exchange.

After two minutes of silence I started analyzing what it was we'd been doing. Us! Relatives who love each other. We'd been playing the "mine is bigger" playschool game. We'd been comparing the incomparable to see who'd had it harder at which time, as if there were a ruler along which this could all be measured, as if we were really set on winning the battle.

I felt degraded, scolded, as all I'd wanted was the chance to bare my soul, to whine about my difficulties. I didn't need help or to be saved. I loved my life the way it was, but this didn't mean that it wasn't damn hard sometimes and that I didn't feel like having a good moan now and again. But it wasn't my aunt's fault. This situation couldn't have come about without my participation. I didn't step out of the exchange by saying "Listen, let's not compare things. I just wanted to have a good moan and that's all. I was just looking for a bit of support." Instead I went into a game I don't like so readily that I only noticed in retrospect that I hadn't enjoyed being in it at all.

When I left the apartment five minutes later, I was feeling grateful for this little episode. I could take something really important from it with me. When my child comes up to me and says, for example, "Mummy, I hate this so much, I have to learn ten verses of this poem by heart, yuck" I'll definitely not react by saying "Don't be funny, only ten verses? I had to learn hundreds of pages of stuff at university." Or when he shares his sadness about being turned down by the girl he likes, perhaps he only wants a hug and not for me to say: "Relax. If your father and I split up with all of you children, now that would really be a catastrophe – but until you have children, it's just a game. It's no biggie." And all this does not actually mean that these sentences are always wrong and cannot be of help in some situations. When my brain is no longer overtaken or ruled by my emotions, after I've had a good cry, all clever remarks, wisdom, and even advice are welcome.

All bugs are insects, but...

All children are sweet when they're sleeping, but not all children are sleeping when they're sweet.

They can't not see a psychologist!

It took me years to not see in my mothering only those areas where there was room for improvement. I needed a good few self-awareness techniques to twist the whip out of my hand, the whip I used to lash myself at the foot of the sculpture of the Ideal Mother. I held on to my former expectations only to the extent that if my children were to see a psychologist one day, the reason wouldn't be that I'd beaten them or that I was an alcoholic. They'll almost certainly see one for some reason or another. And so they should. Self-awareness is an incredibly interesting thing. I don't want to deprive my children of the chance to scream at me, to regress into their embryonic stage in an altered state of consciousness, to blame me for not giving them more attention or for giving them too much of it. What kind of mother would want her children to suffer the experience, while on a voyage of self-discovery, of standing as an outsider, ill at ease, looking at the others immersed in their cry-flow, after a delving-deep exercise, unable to come up with any childhood trauma of their own?

It's your fault

I read more and more often: "Take responsibility for your actions, your decisions; it's your fault, you can do something about it."

I truly believe that I'm responsible for my own life and that I'm the one with the ability to do something about it. Not fate. Not my mother. Not my father. Not my husband. Not God. At the same time, I can see a trap in this view. If I'm not at the stage where I want to make a move for myself, where I want some kind of change, then I can easily turn it against myself: Well, if I'm responsible, then this means that it's my fault! I blame and hurt myself simultaneously, which not only doesn't help, but also pushes me deeper under water.

It's my decision what I decide to use this approach for, whether I let it become a stinging, painful whip in my hands, whether I let it take me towards guilt. If I'm able to accept my faults or look for places to improve, then the same approach can become a surfboard, keeping me on top of the waves of my everyday days.

Robot mum

When I go to do the shopping with the children, even setting off is a fiasco. Imagine this scenario: crying, rushing. Luckily, as I hoped, she falls asleep on the way. At the shop, quickly, quickly into the trolley just what's needed. My fear grows constantly that she'll open her eyes and feel hungry. Then she'll ask, and demand and I'll fall to pieces. But phew, it's done. Everything important is in the trolley. We're at the checkout. I'm putting my things on the conveyor belt... and right then and there she wakes up. And everything I'm afraid of ensues: she's crying, wailing, getting hot in her winter clothes. I want to get the whole thing over and done with, quickly, quickly. Poor thing, my little star, calm down. In a minute, in a minute, in a minute. The child is bright red, I'm burning up. I'd give anything for it to be over as soon as possible, for me to finally be able to feed her. I don't notice that I'm also hungry because I haven't given myself time to have breakfast. I didn't even put an apple in my bag. I'd needed to pee at home, but her crying stressed me out so much that I'd just left. I'm trying to give and give my best. I'm sweating, tearing myself apart. I'm consumed by it all while I imagine I'm doing the right thing because I'm putting her first. And then it all ends up with her crying and me falling to pieces anyway.

So, what could I do differently? If, for example, I notice that I also have needs, that would be great. I could at least recognise that I'll have them at some point because as much as I've tried, I haven't managed to become totally mechanised... yet. I could pretend to be my own child: it would be good to pee before leaving home, too. Like my child, there's a good chance that I'll get hungry during the two-hour project ahead.

And it'd be rather useful to have an extra jumper with me as well, just in case I feel cold at the playground. And if none of this works, then I could remember that I also have a mother I can call and have a cry to. A virtual hug can help me through a difficult situation. Or I could even ask her to do the shopping for me next time.

The smell of freedom

After so much breastfeeding, changing nappies, babbling, getting up in the night, winding, going to the playground, giving knee-rides.... my desire for freedom is so great that it can squash the self-judging me to death – the me who thinks that a good mother is forever loyal to her child, never leaves his side, industriously and incessantly teaches him things; the good mother who lives her life to prove deserving of the good mother scarf. So, I take a deep breath, gather my courage, and go on. It'll be fine. Then I go out to do the shopping ALONE!

Thank yous

"Thank you for looking after them yesterday!" I say to my parents. "Thanks for hanging out the clothes!" I say to my husband. But the question instantly arises in me: why am I saying thanks?!

By doing so, I become a party to something I disagree with. It's not a favour when a grandparent spends time with their grandchildren. I don't owe anyone a debt of gratitude for hanging out the washing unless it was the neighbour who came over to help. However, it still feels right to express the feelings within (for me to give something to them instead of saying thanks) and it's important for them to get something. So, instead of thank you, I could say: "It was reassuring that my kids were here with you while I was working." or "I'm really glad that I got to read for ten minutes instead of hanging out the washing!"

Creativity

Being a parent requires a considerable amount of creativity. And I'm not necessarily thinking about whether I can sew a doll's house out of old socks, but of those moments when the two-year-old has been throwing a professional tantrum for forty-three minutes, or when the nine-year-old argues amazingly well for watching a movie rated 12+, or when the six-year-old demonstrates an impressively tight grip on a sibling's throat. Right there, at that certain point when I begin to feel that I'm losing the battle, that I'm at a crossroads where I let myself lose it all or I find my strength, some hidden source of energy tucked away somewhere on a back-shelf surface and I try to somehow manoeuvre myself out of the given situation. Well, that's where creativity is a must.

It also takes creativity to feed young ones, and the more there are, the more skill is needed. When thinking of everyday cooking or even ordering food in, a complex mathematical formula is presented by trying to aggregate the data produced by the who-eats-what lists, and the task of turning the results into something interesting.

It takes creativity to please – what surprise to get for whom, what to give each of them for a birthday-Christmas-

Hanukkah. We've already got one of those. There are three of these in the house. We've one of those made of wood. We've had one like this before but we hated it. This is brilliant but unfortunately, he doesn't want one; he wants this. I really don't want to listen to the sound it makes. That one would be perfect, but only in two years' time. This one would be the best choice, but how can I find one and can I afford it?

It takes creativity to train children, or preferably not train them but to enjoy a mutual learning process in our years of living together. Generally speaking, it doesn't work for long if I use only one weapon, so cannons, machine guns, crossbows, bombs, slingshots, devil cartridges, and water guns are all tools necessary for achieving my goal.

Whether the child is big or small, getting out of a situation we're stuck in creatively may multiply my energy. When I was going through the colic period with my newborn twins, there were times when I tied a piece of rope to my leg with the other end secured by elastic to the car seat which hung from the ceiling – so while I was feeding one on the sofa, I could rock the other one to sleep using my leg. Thus, I managed to create some relaxed, harmonious cry-free minutes, which is no small feat during the baby period.

There is no weekend when I don't have to rack my brain to find something to do that is interesting for two twelve-year-olds, a ten-year-old, a three-year-old, and an eighteen-month-old, something that is available at the same place and at the same time. If we manage to find something that they all enjoy, then not only are we all recharged, but we've also invested our energy into accumulating good experiences instead of picking on each other.

I don't have much chance of being creative when I'm so tired that my guts are hanging out like shoelaces. I can't create from zero strength. Handling all situations with good humour and calm, creating individual solutions, while remaining patient as I untangle the Gordian knots as expected of a super mum – well, that's an expectation that may be there but, in the end, it'll result in me feeling dissatisfied with myself. Discovering how many small things I have managed to solve creatively can help me strengthen my self-esteem, make me see and appreciate that things are just fine as they are. And naturally, if I wish to, I can make them even better – luckily there are 218 opportunities that present themselves every day for me to improve my creativity rate.

Rubbish days

I can feel in the morning if it's going to be a rubbish day: I don't have the strength to get over the night I spent breastfeeding; I can't see any good aspects to not having slept more than three hours at any time for the past three years; I'm an impatient, shouting, unlikeable character. I can feel that I'm unable to pull myself together and drag myself out of the hole: I'm unfair to everybody, with no fresh ideas, but no matter how hard I try to be proactive, it just doesn't work. The children can sense that the day is the devil's, so tension mounts higher than usual in them, too.

On such days, there are three things I can do. I can switch into the "do no harm" mode. In essence, this means that I shouldn't try to be good, I should just try not to do harm. I give them food, but I don't want to cook anything amazing. Pizza will do. I don't want to think of anything interesting to do for everyone. I accept that sometimes it's okay if the older kids watch a movie while I go around the corner to the nearest playground with the little ones. I'm afraid to use the easy options because I'm afraid of my own judgement: that I'm not good enough. If I lose the extremes, it becomes much better – instead of thinking that I'm never good enough, it's much better to say that today, I can't do any better than this. And tomorrow is another day.

On rubbish days, it's an even better solution to remove myself altogether from my family and leave my children with someone who has more to give. Meanwhile I can also recharge, regenerate.

And then there's the third option: to be glad about every minute that brings me closer to the end of the day.

With force

When, let's say, my son would like to wade into the ice-cold water of Lake Balaton. When he decides to assume a horizontal position in a dangerous place, for example in the middle of a triple-lane road. Or when he's screaming at the top of his lungs because he'd like to listen to different music while I am driving, and I'm ready to go off my head from the frustration of powerlessness knowing it's not exactly ideal to drive in this state. Or when I ask him nicely, but words are of no use, we can't get past whatever it is and move on, then I'm not efficient if I don't sort the emergency promptly. Sometimes I have to use methods and techniques that are not my favourites. For example, force. I can pick him up and move him or set the boundary with my voice or tone. And I get to bear the consequences, such as guilt, with dignity. And then, when the emergency is over, I can start thinking about what I can possibly do differently next time. Though it's also okay to be glad about being successful in averting danger and avoiding corporal punishment, for example, which is drastically against my value system.

Today versus tomorrow

I find it easier to notice where and what could be changed for a better and smoother life than to see things that are already wonderful in it. Apart from my own life, I'm responsible for the lives of five children, so there are many areas in which things could be chiselled, further refined. The wish to make everyone's life happier every single day creates an ongoing desire to do some work within. Some find it hard to make a shift in themselves and see what they could do for their children's happiness. The most difficult thing for me is to keep focusing on how great things are already, that the sun came up today and that my children are so funny, that my husband and I are in love, that the salami hasn't gone off.

I like about myself that I search for and take steps to be happy. And sometimes this step is immobility: I'm learning to slow down the present, to look at the now, to see how wide the given realm is. I enjoy not making a habit of walking past the achievements of the day (everyone having clean socks for the day again, for instance), the joys (it's spring, no big coats and boots, leaving home thirty-two kilos lighter) and the drops of happiness (laughing together, hugs, exciting adolescent conversations) without noticing them.

Problem

Who is to sit where in the car is a constant problem in my family. There are less-preferred seats. There are children who can sit in the front. There are ones who cannot sit in the back, because it's important for me to be able to reach for the millet ball he's pushed up his nose instead of his mouth while I'm driving. There was an arrangement whereby everyone sat in a different place for every journey. There was a rotation system in place with a weekly change. There were so many other things. But the fighting remained.

"Why is it me again who has to climb in?"

"Why is it me again who sits next to so and so?"

"Why is it him again sitting in the front when he sat there the time before...?!"

I tried explaining that this problem is nothing compared to the fact that there's a war going on in Syria, but they weren't really touched by this. I tried going into detail about how hard us adults are working so we'll be able to buy another car that we can all fit in comfortably, but this didn't bring roaring results either. I tried being really strict, but even I didn't like that.

For now, I've passed the problem-solving over to them. Let them figure out something that suits everyone. Well, we'll see. One thing is for sure, I'm less frustrated as a result of passing on the problem-solving task, and they're excited that there is a task – so there's no solution yet but the situation is better already.

Who is high-risk?

At twenty weeks, at my first ultrasound scan, it turned out that I was expecting twins. The worries came from the outside that I should feel I have a high-risk pregnancy while I was feeling better than ever before. No nausea. No extreme tiredness. My blood sugar and my blood pressure and all my other measurable and immeasurable indicators were perfect. A little on my high horse, I saw myself as someone who wasn't at all phased by the first twelve weeks. No matter how much the hospital, the health visitor, the books, and my relatives tried to make me out to be high-risk, no matter how much passion they used to try to scare me about twin births, expecting and giving birth to my twins was the smoothest run of them all. Similarly, with my third kid, I enjoyed the first twelve weeks carefree and then the next twenty-eight without any scares.

And then came my fourth child and I found out what the hormonal express of the first twelve weeks is really like. Changing moods? Like a pendulum on a crane, that's what it's like. I realised in a schizoid manner with delays of a few minutes that oops, I'd just been crying and that it was me who was shouting five seconds ago. Why was I moved to tears by a frankfurter commercial? I couldn't even keep up with myself. I admired my husband for having stuck with me, so far. I, myself, found it hard to live with me. I think I can safely say that I was a pregnant woman presenting a high risk to others.

Slower minutes, longer hours

I love the end bit so much. None of my children were born

before the fortieth week. There was one who came out in the forty-second, so I know that there's a fair bit of tension in this last period of waiting. And yet these days or weeks toward the end are like nothing I've experienced in any other area or at any other time of my life. They could have ended in as little as two hours in a way that I could never go back to the same place. It was also possible, though, that it could have lasted for weeks yet. Slower minutes and longer hours shaped me physically and emotionally. I got used to this constant transformation that became a motionless eternity at the same time. It felt unimaginable that my pregnancy would ever be any different. I was both looking forward to and dreading the end – if not the birth itself, definitely the unknown. While at the same time it was unbelievably exciting that within a few hours I would be living with somebody I'd never seen before.

Happy childhood?

Let's go back to the beginning of life. First, there's a world a good few degrees colder than the one before. Food no longer comes on a cord. Hugs are only given when others want to give them. Lights are blindingly strong. Something cold is placed on my bum. I can't get the eyelash out of my eye. I can't reach the interesting, colourful bits. I have to wait years to be able to climb on those much-wanted things.

Then I'm put among twenty-five other similar beings whom I fight with for objects, and the love and attention of one or two people. Then the same thing at home, fighting against the incomprehensible brushing of teeth and bedtime. My siblings frequently push me over, hit me, take what's mine, for example, my mum's lap. I'm not allowed to eat as much chocolate as I'd like, it's supposed to be unhealthy, even though I don't understand what the word means. And that's another thing. There's a whole load of things I don't understand.

At school, the children and the teachers judge me, I try to live up to their expectations with all my strength. I squirm at the start of the year-opening ceremony in my white shirt in thirty-five degrees during the awfully boring speech by the headmaster. If my breasts start growing at the age of eleven, that's a problem. If they don't, that's not nice either. For the contemporary group not to shut me out, I must magically create a perfect hairdo every morning and my clothes must also be fancied by the other kids. I'd be glad if I didn't have to decide on a school trip in high school, whether to have a puff of the cool kids' cigarettes behind the wooden shed or admit that not one bit of me feels like smoking.

Good grades, entrance exams – I've to think well ahead in primary school. Choosing a career at the very end of my childhood? Hmm. I'm looking forward to a more peaceful, more tension-free, happier adulthood.

Dying of exhaustion on the road to an ideal motherhood

At some point in the past I used to think that I'd be a good mother if all my attention was focused on my children, if I spent all my time with them – but no, that's certainly not the case. What they need more than anything is a happy mother. A mother who's able to give. The quantity is important, but the quality is of far more significance. If I run out of me, what have I got left to give? If I become grey, how can I make their world colourful? If I switch to survivor mode, focused on fulfilling my duties as a robot and so become emotionally unavailable, how can they safely attach to me?

My oldest, my twin sons, suffered from colic; they almost never slept at the same time for six months. I was either putting one or the other to sleep. I was feeding them one after the other, day and night, rocking their butts incessantly. They were about five or six months old when one afternoon my mother popped in and, looking at my mop-like face, asked me if I'd had two minutes to spend on my own that day. I looked at her uncomprehendingly: how and when? One of them is always crying, requiring something from me, wanting some of me?! Put them in their bed, go outside, take a few deep breaths, and recharge for a minute or two! And if they're crying, think that it's great; at least you can hear from a distance that they're working well.

It took me till after having my fourth child to understand I was doing this instinctively; I was able to take this piece of advice, free of guilt. Sometimes I'm still devastated by motherhood, but because I know I can function differently as well, it does not crush me any more.

Early imprinting

Newly hatched ducklings and baby geese start following the first moving thing bigger than them that they see. The connection that forms between thirteen and sixteen hours after birth cannot be changed later. Whatever was imprinted then, that's the mother, and that's that, be that a real duck or the boots of Konrad Lorenz.* Luckily, with the human child there's no such thing that we've only got a few hours for – if I can't breastfeed at the beginning, I can keep trying for weeks even. If I'm not able to find the mother in me who's capable of providing safety for my baby immediately, I've hours to look for her every day. If I'm going through a difficult life phase, if there are a few weeks or months when I'm more tired, more tense, more impatient than usual, I've many, many years to self-correct. It's great that we're not ducks, that we have hands, and in them we hold the possibility to make changes.

One by one

When difficulties swell into mountains, it's chilling to even think of them. Something my midwife mother once told me during labour helps me a lot: "You don't have to survive the whole birth, just get through one contraction at a time." When I'm struggling with imaginary or real mountains that seem to be impossible to climb in any case, I get on more easily if I don't focus on the distance ahead or look at the faraway peak, but focus on my feet as I take my steps. You don't have to bring them all up, you don't have to get through it all, only this minute, this hour, this day.

---

* Konrad Lorenz – an Austrian ethologist, Nobel prize winner. He studied imprinting in geese, who bond with the first moving object they see within the first hours of hatching.

3

Reshaping the patterns that shape us

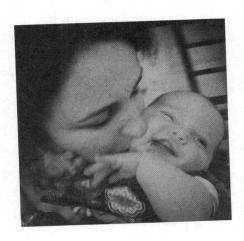

When I realise that I try to direct my kids toward the right path the same way my mother used to do with me: a spoonful of reasoning, a spoonful of indulgence, a pinch of craftiness, and a teaspoonful of psychology with as much love as it'll soak up; when I'm being playful or funny or impatient using exactly the same words and actions as my father used to use with me; when I exhale through my mouth as my grandfather used to do when we wore him down; when I'm able to talk to my kids in the same patient and reassuring tone as my mother does to me; when I care for them with food and love the way my grandmother used to care for me; when I decide to do something totally differently to my elders but for some reason I end up doing the very same...

I don't need to dig down to my roots. I don't need to see my parts hidden underground in order for me to operate. Digging is dirty and mostly hard work, but I still like it. On the one hand, it's interesting – there are many treasures to be found under the ground – on the other hand, it pays off a thousand-fold to make a change to things I dislike in my own life.

The language of patterns

Patterns are like our mother tongue. We live our days with them for umpteen years. They don't require direct learning, they automatically and invisibly sink in and define us. If my mother and my father frequently kiss each other happily and regularly hold one another, this becomes normal to me. I learn the movement, the gestures, the act itself and it isn't strange for me to do the same in my daily life; I'll express my love in this way as well. If there's no tactility in the family, no kisses, no hugs, then such expressions of love will seem alien to me. This may mean that I'll have no great desire for such displays of affection, but it may also mean that it'll be a priority for me to find a partner who is a tactile, cuddly person, who displays bodily affection freely, as I have a deficiency in this area. A pattern, just like a language, is not good or bad. Patterns are Lego blocks with which I can build anything I want, and I can also rebuild things any time I feel like. It might seem like I've a given number of blocks, but I can also recognise that the world is full to the brim with pieces suitable for expansion.

Just like a fairytale

As well as patterns of behaviour brought from home, we're also unconsciously influenced by norms defined by social expectations.

I don't really know any poems or fairytales where love is not depicted as some kind of extreme concept, where it's not described as a co-dependent/addictive relationship:

"Without you I shall die!"

"You are my everything! I'm nothing without you; I'm worthless."

"If you leave me, I'll die of sorrow!"

"And they lived happily ever after."

Love is what we burn in and what we die of; love lasts till we die. We're fed daily with poems and stories, unnoticed, from a young age until these become our norms. It's as if the kind of love where I don't depend on another, where I exist as a separate entity, love that I don't die from, doesn't really exist. And what do we do when we grow out of childhood? We try so hard to live up to these norms, and search for the ideal one. We may even find them, but if we're not able to keep the flames going, we feel that either we or they have made a mistake. Either way, what we have is bad. They're bad or we're bad, but something is definitely bad, as we're not living the perfect copy of the love we internalised and imagined as ideal.

What would happen if we just changed the end of those stories to "and they lived together for as long as they were both happy"?!

The root of my workings

It's a difficult evening. Picture the scene: there are tensions, potholes on the road to bed. She finally reaches for her pillow but it's dirty and this really sets her off. I consider this testing of my boundaries as below the belt. I feel angry. I didn't save enough strength for this episode. I've run out of patience. That's enough. Sleep time and that's that. She must be sensing my weakness as she goes straight for the jugular: she wails uncontrollably. Well, all right, I haven't just started parenting either. It's time to set boundaries right now, I'm thinking. I tell her that it's not okay to scream like that at this time of night because the schoolchildren must have their rest. She doesn't give a damn. It's making me angrier and angrier, my nerves are in tatters, I'm falling apart. After a brief self-assessment, I tell her that I have the patience to ask nicely only one more time and then I'll start screaming as well, for I have no more strength, no place to recharge. Like kissing the dead. I lose it and pick her up, take her into the study and shut the door on her. I can feel, I know, that this is terribly inept, but I also feel that this is the best I can do right now, and all my other solutions at the moment are much worse than this. She's crying relentlessly, wailing, while I'm trying to take deep breaths on the other side of the door to calm down somehow and find some tiny trace of strength in me to enable me to pull our suffocating selves out onto the shore. I take a deep breath, go in, hug her, talk to her, make a deal, take her back to bed. She falls asleep.

The next afternoon sees yet another terrible outburst, because I fail to ask her which particular pair of shoes she'd like to wear. I just take out a pair I consider suitable. More fool me. A blast of tension erupts from her, unstoppable, her hormones are screaming and what does she do? She marches into the study and shuts the door on herself. And there I stand, astounded. This is how the way we work evolves. My mother shuts me in the room one night and from the following day I shut myself in. Phew, that's rough.

Mechanisms that work

When my mother was in prison, we, the members of the family, all coped differently with the trauma. In that period, I created one of my favourite pieces of work to this day, a video series entitled *56 pajamas*. When I was working, I was able to shut out everything else. I operated in a detached, exclusive mode. I didn't allow any pain, worry, fear, or shudders to get through, for they could squash me to death if I didn't lock them out airtight – through the eye of a needle a whole mountain of pain could pour into me.

Meanwhile, I walked the road of self-knowledge. I'd just started a coaching course that would last a few years. We were studying and experiencing directly for ourselves how crying helped in processing, accepting, and moving on. "Has your grandmother had a good cry yet?" I'm asked by a friend. "No, my grandmother hasn't had a good cry yet." I look at my grandmother watching her fifty-five-year-old daughter on the news in handcuffs and leg irons. And she's not crying. So, somehow, she should be given help to cry, says the girl. Help to cry? My grandmother lost her mother when she was nine months old. Her grandmother, the person who brought her up, died in a wagon on the way to a concentration camp. Her father dropped dead when they were liberated. She was seventeen then. She lost her husband at the age of fifty-two. And now she's looking at her daughter in leg irons. I don't know if I could survive even half such trauma, not to mention survive the way she's survived. She's healthy and well, unbelievably well accomplished. She's been a cheerful and amazing grandmother to me all my life. Not on one single occasion has she made the choice to step away from her pain, with a suicide attempt, for instance. When we asked her during the imprisonment period how she was feeling, she gave a mantra-like answer: "Physically well, emotionally poorly." She said she would cry when her daughter was released. Because you can't break down on the road, only when the horror is all over. She has a tried and tested survival method, so why should I take it from her? Why should I get her to cry just because I think that it's the healthy way to release and process pain? I'm rather envious, actually. I wish I had such a brilliant protective shield. Now that I've written this, I realise that I must have taken a leaf out of my grandmother's book – it was me who was there when my mother, reduced to skin and bone, was led out in shackles in court and it didn't cross my mind for a second to cry.

Small kids, small problems; big kids, big problems?

Small kids, small problems; big kids, big problems. I've heard this saying from my mother and many others so many times that for years I didn't even question it. I didn't feel small kids were a small problem; instead, I was dreading that as they grew, the problems would grow with them.

Now that my children are older, I think it's a better survival mechanism to either see the period we've already successfully come through as the bigger problem, or I would simply not even try to compare it to the challenges of the coming years. So, I've reinterpreted and rephrased the saying to: *Smaller kids – fewer types of problems; bigger kids – a wider range of problems.* The difficulties of a newborn tend to be in the area of hungry-tired-pooey-peey-windy-insecure and a mixture of these, while the bigger they are the more refined, crafted, and complex their needs and desires become, and so do my tasks with them.

If I think back to the period when I was at home with three

under-threes, I don't see that as any easier than now, when there's a small one and a smaller one and some teenagers in my family. In fact, sometimes I think it's a miracle I survived the period with three small children without going mad. And, of course, I can't say that I've survived the adolescent period yet, as for the next fifteen to eighteen years there's always going to be someone in that phase in my family, so I see shifting things within my own head, instead of the constant struggling and whining about how difficult it is as my only survival option.

F*!^ you, great-grandmother!

The everyday psychology hype of the past decade has taken us from blaming fate and the state for our lives to blaming our parents. I smoke because my mother didn't breastfeed me for long enough. I smoke because my father shouted at me once with a cigarette in his hand. I could have become a pianist had my mother not forced the violin on me. I have become a pianist because my father pushed for the violin. It's become a cool thing to know how much influence our childhood patterns and events bring to bear on the way we operate at present. And this gives an impetus to slide over into blaming our parents for everything. We can lean back, we have a scapegoat.

There's some sort of luscious sensation in blaming my parents. Because this is an incredibly easy way of removing my own responsibility from it all. If it's my mother's and/or my father's fault, it can't be mine.

If they are, indeed, the cause of my failings, they must also be the reason for the things I like about myself. They're to be held responsible for me altogether. When my mother lists the areas she feels she was not good in, it doesn't feel nice. I like myself the way I am, which is also a direct result of what she was like with me. The moments she considers bad have shaped me as much as those she has placed in the "well-done" box. When she cracks the whip at the mother she's been to me, it feels like I'm a spoiled sculpture.

There's a desired father and a desired mother image in me, the kind of parents I'd like to have had. I would've wished for more of their time and attention. I wouldn't have chosen to go to crèche at the age of seven months, and I would like to have had parents who could live together happily. Just like in a fairytale, I'd like to have been the fruit of the prince and princess's love. And there I get stuck. I often go back to grieve for my unlived childhood. It's like being stuck in a certain stage of bereavement.

What can possibly take me forward? One of the things, for example, is if I talk to my parents or tell them that it would've been good if... The deposited layer of dirt can thus be washed off and then I can move on in the bereavement process toward acceptance. Maybe it doesn't happen immediately on my first attempt, but if I keep trying, we can make a connection on which a new type of relationship can be built between us. It's possible to do this even if our parents are not alive; it's liberating to express such feelings just to ourselves.

They won't be able to help anyway. If I don't want to or can't move on, they may apologise a thousand times, but I'll stay stuck. Nobody can take a step with my feet and no one can shift my inner parts either.

For that matter, essentially my ancestors are responsible for everything. My grandmother didn't love my father in a way that could've made him a perfect father for me, so it's all down to my grandmother. Surely my grandmother was not loved by her mother for her to have been able to become the person that would have made it possible for my father to be the person who would have been good for me, so f*!^ my great-grandmother as well. Not to mention great-grandfathers. Okay, there goes the anger phase, so I can slowly move toward acceptance and the appreciation and re-evaluation of those things that were actually given.

Then I get to the stage when I can actually do something with everything I've been given. And just what I decide to do with it is up to me alone. If I don't shift the responsibility, I can make quite attractive parents for myself. The shortfall is slowly and gradually reduced, the good sides stand out, the warming memories come forth, and I'm flooded with pictures of my childhood when my mother and my father enriched my life with so much, with so many different kinds of love. And simultaneously, as the old goodness appears, in my present I notice all those much-loved parts of me, inside and out, all those qualities and the value system I also want to pass on to my own children and I understand that it was all given to me by them. And should I still come upon bits of me I dislike, I can be like Cindy Crawford, and turn my large birthmark from a blemish into an advantage.

Divorce

For years I believed that my parents' divorce was a bad thing because it hurt me. I hated that they didn't stay together, that I missed my father a lot, that I hated my mother's new partner. Then, gradually and slowly, I began to see why it was so very good that they had got divorced. When I remember their fights – well, if I'd had to listen to those for years, I'd rather have swallowed fifty centipedes a day. For a long time, I was able to take strength from their divorce, set on doing better myself, not wanting to follow that path. It helped me look for solutions to my relationship problems as I struggled to save my children from experiencing the splitting up of their parents. Then, when I could no longer find a reason for struggling on, it was my parents' divorce that helped me yet again to understand that there was life after a divorce and that I could find my happier self and trust that I was not doing harm to but doing right by my children. Everything can be used in support of something and its complete opposite as well.

Bedwetting

I wet the bed until the age of eleven. As a child, I walked the warrior's path of methods to break the habit. Sometimes I wasn't allowed to drink after 6pm, and I'd try to suck the water out of my toothbrush. At times I had to eat five egg yolks from the afternoon to the evening. I still don't like egg yolks much. I travelled to Budapest from Szeged to see psychologists. One of them believed in writing a diary: if I didn't wet myself, I was to draw a sun for the given day; if I did wet the bed, I was to draw a cloud. The thing I referred to as "the fire equipment," which was clipped to my pajama top on one end and secured with snap buttons in between my legs in a way that one wire ran underneath my pajamas, and the other on top, was the most terrifying gadget. When I peed myself, and it got wet, the circuit closed, and it started screaming like the siren of a fire engine. None of the strategies worked. I wet the bed relentlessly. The psychologists and my parents had given up on me when, a few years later, I stopped by myself.

Twenty years later a little girl was born into the family. She wet herself to the age of three, then four, then five, then six. I asked her father whether he was worried, whether he wanted to take her to see a psychologist or someone else.

"The best thing for her is if I simply leave her alone and she'll stop when she's ready. I learnt from your example."

I wouldn't remove the trials and tribulations of bedwetting from my life, but I couldn't see a good side to them for ages. I carried something for a long time, so it didn't have to be carried by someone else – and thus I'm fine with it.

Useless objects?

To this very day it's a sore point for me that my mother chucked out the doll's buggy I loved so much. With my adult mind I understand that it was bashed up, shabby, with the wheels barely moving and it also had a hole in it, but still I didn't see a single thing wrong with it back then. I loved it, just the way it was. And what good has this awful trauma brought me? A few years ago, when moving flat, I didn't want to be the judge of what was important to which child of mine, so I allowed them to decide whether they wanted to keep an old chewing gum or a footless soldier, as the former might be a memory, the latter a perfect corpse. I was afraid that they would find all their knick-knacks useful, but this wasn't what happened. They selected quite surprising things as ready to be passed on to children in need. And yes, there were some things I would've considered useless that moved with us into the new flat and well, so what, half a kilo of it is produced daily (and simultaneously half a kilo of stuff that's important disappears). And I must admit, a few things that I thought were valuable, and the kids pronounced ready for the bin, I ended up keeping.

Handovers

I hand over the hanging out of the washing. They hate it. I hand over the taking out of the rubbish. They hate it. They pair socks reluctantly. They like being with their younger siblings provided it's not considered looking after them. What chores do they do happily? More or less nothing... if it's a chore. As I don't want them to do nothing, I must think of something.

At times I have the energy to make things into a game. We've had a sock-pairing competition, experiencing all the joy and excitement of every second. However, I don't always have the creative energy to figure out how to ask for help playfully.

Their recurrent problem is to respond with "OK, but what about the others?" Is his brother going to hang out the washing as well? "It's easier to hang out the washing than to do the washing up." "But why don't you ever ask him to do anything?" To prevent such comments, I write the chores on small pieces of paper and they have to take one – fate is then blamed for all the injustice, instead of me.

It happens that when listing all tasks, I ask them to come to an agreement about what's agreeable to each of them, which ones they're each willing to do – I also feel more like tidying up than putting clothes away sometimes. I try to make my requests varied: please put away 17 things before evening. For some reason, this works better than asking them to tidy up.

To avoid misunderstandings, I tell them that I don't hang

out the washing twice a day because I enjoy doing it so much. "Then why do you do it?" one of them asks. I've never thought about it, so I'm glad of the question. Because by keeping house, I look after them, us. Tidying up, cleaning, providing food and clean clothes are all things I give every single day. They're the small daily presents from me to them. I'd like them to notice and appreciate these and experience themselves that it's no easy ride.

I know, I can see that my fixations and my patterns imprinted on my bones have an effect on my behaviour. I grew up with my mum earning the money and taking care of the household and the children as well. My aunt and my grandmother were both amazed by how decent my mother's partner was for taking the rubbish out twice a week. It was the norm in my family that the women should be strong as a bull and work their guts out on all fronts while falling at the feet of their partners with a heart filled with gratitude if the men took on as little as a thousandth of all the chores. I'd like to have had a different division of labour in my male-female relationships and the point of change was not at "I'll find a decent man one day", but at working hard on myself to move away from the idea that I can only be a fine woman if I'm stronger and tougher than everyone, especially my partner. I've learnt to let go of and hand over some tasks and, as a result, in my family the man-woman/father-mother model is not what I've brought with me from home. Out of the sack that hides a thousand small different tasks, from taking care of small children to earning money, there are very few which I don't share with my husband. And with all this, I've still managed to remain a woman who's as strong as a bull.

My mother tried not to put any burden on us, her children, either. So, when I moved out and had to take care of my own home before having children, I remember the feeling when I realised, oh my God, if it's like this, she had so much to do every single day. I felt angry that she didn't involve me, that I had to realise in retrospect how hard it must have been for her when we were living together. I could have done things to make it easier on her. Of course, it's also quite possible that she did ask me a thousand times and I just failed to hear her.

Simultaneously, I feel that while I'd like to hand over some chores to the kids, I don't want to overload them. For example, it can't happen that we don't go out somewhere at the weekend until they clean their rooms, or that everyone must do something to help every day. I try to consider their individual loads as well: if one gets home from school at 1pm, he can be given a heavier load than the one who gets home at 4pm and starts training at 5pm. This is nothing but injustice for the one who got home earlier, of course. OK, I take responsibility. Life is unfair, but the tables will turn and in the long term, it's all justly unfair.

Then, there's also the thing that in the short term, handing things over and asking for help often makes things harder rather than easier. It's so much easier to put away the Duplo than convince the two-year-old to help. It's so much easier to tidy up their desks than to ask the teenagers ten times. But slowly the time will come when they tidy up their own rooms without being asked, when they'll come and help me when I'm putting things away, when they'll put their own plates into the dishwasher. And when they see that I'm dead beat they'll come and ask: "Mama, can I help you with anything?"

Idol

I'm small, 115cm tall. I can remember the place in the corridor of our flat in Szeged where in my mind's eye, I'm standing with my mother. I'm looking up at that beautiful slim woman and I'm listening to why she's drinking that horrible-smelling stuff and how the apple vinegar diet works. There and then I'm learning about dieting from my idol, acquiring how not to like my beautiful slim self, learning to make my body suffer and hurt.

I've put tons of self-knowledge hours into untangling my body image disorder. It wasn't only this incident I found, there were more treasures in the box such as trainee teachers at school making comments about my breasts, or a man masturbating next to me on the 4/6 tram – being a woman is a dangerous thing! My father called me Fatty until I was twelve, which I simply loved because there was so much love in it.

I'm not saying that looking into the mirror today I feel infinitely satisfied, but I spend only half the time that I used to spend chewing that bone. I don't believe that I'll see myself as perfect at any point in the future, but that's no longer my aim either. If I can be the mother (= idol) to my daughter who doesn't torment her own body but starts doing exercise if she considers herself fat and we can enjoy eating together, well, that's good enough for me.

Once, when I'd just finished having a bath, she was standing by, handing me my clothes. As I put my knickers on, she said: "Mummy, you really do have a big bum." This made me laugh so hard, it was so immensely liberating to realise that I no longer keep saying this to myself.

Invaluable

My mother worked as a gynecologist-obstetrician in a hospital for seventeen years. She never accepted gratitude money, she never accepted a single envelope.* She hadn't worked at the clinic for ages, when one day, I must have been about fifteen, we were sitting in the kitchen mulling over the fact that we couldn't afford to go on holiday. That was when I first heard her say that perhaps she should have done things differently, maybe she'd made a mistake. She should have accepted all those envelopes as it would make and would have made life so much simpler. How much better we would be living now and how much better we would have been able to live in the meantime. We could be going on holidays several times each year. She could have bought her children flats, mansions, or palaces. Even as a teenager longing for holidays, clothes, and hi-fi systems, I was still able to reply instantly that she'd given me much more by her model of integrity, by never accepting money, by living the way she believed right. No amount of money could possibly buy me a verbally and practically clear and coherent value system, a point of reference and strength for my entire life.

About snot

Snot is thought of as a bad thing: disgusting, infectious. Don't pick it, don't wipe it on anything, don't eat it. Seen in a different light, it's a useful self-defence mechanism. Multifunctional, the body can change its ingredients according to its momentary function: transparent, watery snot helps keep the airways moist, while green snot serves as

---

* In Hungary, patients or their families often give money and/or gifts to their doctors in the hope of getting better treatment or as a way of saying thanks. This custom came about partly because of the low salaries doctors receive. Obstetricians are often given fairly large sums of money by parents after a birth. Although this is a widely accepted practice and known by all, the money is often passed discreetly in an envelope.

a defence against bacilli. We produce between one and one and a half litres of snot a day, unnoticed, most of which we swallow without ever thinking about it.

We don't think about all the old reflexes and learned behavioural patterns that guide us, either. Like snot watering our airways, our reflexes help us choose the ways we act and proceed in the many hundreds of situations we encounter daily. Snot becomes unpleasant from the point at which there is too much of it. It overflows, it cannot be swallowed any more, it stops being unnoticeable, it has to be wiped off, it irritates, it hurts our nose. We can't smell, we can't taste, our voice changes. And we're not too attractive either with green snot running out of our nose. Our reflexes can become the same when they no longer help us, when they stop us from working more freely and smoothly. A blocked nose is just like an inner block – whether we're making a decision or solving a problem or in a path-seeking phase. Self-knowledge work is analogous with a good blowing of the nose. Some experience it as unpleasant, and sometimes it is unpleasant. You can be helped in the process or you can do it yourself. The main thing is the state that follows – we can breathe freely, we can smell again, food has taste again, we'll be carefree and well.

If I suck snot down my throat, it seems like I'm going in the right direction, the mucous doesn't come out, but it can cause a problem elsewhere. For example, it may result in sinusitis. The process of suppressing works the same way – pressure mounts, grievance grows, anxiety increases – and this can create more serious illnesses in our bodies as well as greater blocks in our souls. The accumulated stuff is emptied somewhere, if not necessarily through an illness. For example, unrelieved tension creates anger, which often pours out at unexpected times and in an uncontrolled form.

Everyone has snot. No one has an immaculate nose. If I recover from flu, it doesn't make me immune to snot for the rest of my life. We're snotty kids to our death and a good priest blows his nose to his dying day.

Hair clips

I can barely wait for her hair to grow long enough so I can use hair clips and hairbands. After three sons, I'm bursting with desire to put thousands of little bits in my daughter's hair. She doesn't let me. She can feel that, just like a hungry dog by the dinner table, I'm anxiously waiting for a small bite to drop. I try nice words, requests, reason, force, any which way I can think of, to no avail. "Well, later then, perhaps at nursery, with other children her age, when she sees her friends," other mothers of daughters comfort me. That's a bloody long time away! I buy her hair stuff with kittens, purple ones, glittery ones. She leaves them in her hair for two or three minutes – and I consider this too expensive a sport. I feel hard done by that I cannot fulfill my girlie hair-clip dreams, so I start putting all these lovely bits in my own hair, not having anything better to do with them. And then she comes and takes them from my hair and starts putting them into her own. My words and my clever tricks are defeated by the example I give, no matter how small that example is.

Is there another way?

My mother often said to me throughout my stormy teenage years: "If you carry on like this, we won't get on." And we didn't get on. As far as I can remember, we argued through my entire adolescence.

Is there another way? I've no other pattern to follow. I wasn't living with my father at the time and I didn't have much connection with him either. I would like this to be different with my kids. This is a conscious decision, but is that enough for actually stepping out of what I learnt, of what I know? Is it enough to find a way I'm not familiar with and if that way does exist, is it viable for me?

Why is it useful for me at all that there's this adolescent thing which is already loaded with a bunch of adjectives, such as crazy and scary, even before it arrives? It surely serves me to become more distant, more detached, so that I find it easier to let my growing child go. Why would I move away if it was perfectly harmonious to be with him? When my relationship with someone is rocky, no matter how much I love them, it's my basic instinct to separate. To blame only him for moving further away while I'm right there regardless is much easier. It's hard to admit to myself that I'd be fine with distancing myself from him; a good mother (in my mind) is one who's always there for her children, whether it rains or shines, or the child is an adolescent. But what if I don't always want to be there for him? What if I'd like him to feel safe but I don't always want to be his main source of security? What if I'd like him to find security within instead of through me? Because inner security will be there even when I'm not and it's really far safer for him than relying on me.

And is this possible without us arguing, without us picking on each other, without us falling out? I have no idea, but it's certain that I'm searching vigorously for possibilities – in me.

Good weather

I love the rain. The way it smells, the way it feels, the way it sounds. The way it can change my mood. In theory, rain is bad weather, that's what the meteorologists, the Internet, the standard language says. The fact that I love it does not mean that I can't use the term good weather to mean warm weather, which I personally don't like all that much. If I didn't use these expressions conventionally, I couldn't speak the same language as the majority of people and I don't want to exclude myself. It also makes things simple: I won't always explain that "To me, good weather means when it's raining but now it's warm and sunny so don't put any tights on." No need for tights, the weather is good.

My mother is also fond of rain. I probably learnt to love it from her. And I'm passing on that pattern: we walk in the rain and downpours with the children. Even if they don't necessarily like it later, they already know that rainy weather is the best. Especially for jumping in puddles.

Perseverance or seeking desires?

In my family, my brother was the creative, clever, rhapsodic child who started all sorts of things but didn't complete anything. I can instantly think of four sports that he stopped within a few weeks of starting. I was the hard-working, persevering girl – the not-too-special but user-friendly child. I thought that I was better than him, at least at seeing things through, even if I didn't have as many brains as he did.

When my own children brought the question into my life of whether they should switch sports and whether I should support them in their decision or push for perseverance, only then did I discover new aspects to this question.

First it was swimming. They trained regularly for a few years, won everything, got bored. Before setting off to train, they started asking "Do we have to go today?" We completed the month we had paid for; the year came to an end, and they were done with it. OK, but they needed to do something because all that testosterone regularly exploded in the middle of the room, and I'm not really good at putting up with more than five minutes of fighting a day with a calm Buddha mind. Sport does help there. And so, the true love, ice-hockey, arrived. For years they guzzled, devoured, gorged themselves on it joyously, no matter how much time it took. Irrespective of the number of hours I had to spend standing at the side of the ice rink – at times pregnant, at times with a small baby – their joy compensated unequivocally. The hockey puck became their baby sister's teething ring and instead of stairs she learned to climb my goalkeeper son's kneepads. Her fourth word was "Let's go!" After a few years, the questions began:

"Mama, must we go today?"

"Of course, I like going but..."

"The training is fine but..."

"I like the coach but..."

They didn't have a problem with anything in particular; there was nothing wrong with their tenacity, they just fell out of love with it all. It's the middle of the season, it's a team sport, we can't leave the others in the lurch, we must stick with it at least till the end of the season. But we don't have to stick to this alone, let's look around and see what else is out there, like fencing or floorball. We kept looking at them on the Internet, or in real life. They were happy to try themselves in other sports. I could support them in their search to find what they wanted to do: Let's be happy that we've already enjoyed a few years doing the sport of our dreams and let's believe we can find something similar. They needed six months to find it. Despite the difficulties, I could see in the process how great it was that they didn't stop searching until they found the same feelings they had once had for ice hockey.

It wasn't always as simple as it sounds here, written down. For example, fencing suited them so well, I'd have loved for them to choose that sport. And they seemed to be very gifted, according to the masters. I had to force myself to hold back from pushing them too much in that direction.

As I used to be the persevering and orderly one in the family, inside I had to unwrap the myth that the only right way was to finish what I'd started. Through my children's search for a sport, I was able to put my brother into a different box. I got to understand him and my family's labelling to a greater extent. So how is it then? If you're searching for your desire, you're not persevering because you feel the taste of a number of things? I hope that my children will do everything for only a few weeks, if their gut feeling doesn't take them any further. I hope that they'll persevere in not sticking with anything that takes more than it gives. So, I cheer them on to keep looking for their desires and when they find them, to hold on to them. I don't think members of my family have started to scratch the "he just starts everything" label off my brother, even though, just staying on the subject of sport, he's been doing kung fu for 25 years.

Nothing is ever good enough for you

"Nothing is ever good enough for you." I heard this a lot as a child and I've been reproached in a relationship with the same words. And it is so, indeed. I like to pinpoint desires and goals and fight for them. I like to get ahead according to my own measures and take steps. Well, not always ahead, but sometimes to the left or to the right. And it's true that being in the present is equally important. It makes my life more colourful when I can experience in its completeness what the moment has to give. The two do not exclude one another: At times I can be well in the present, and simultaneously feel what more I desire.

Just look at little Suzy

When I was young, I heard from my grandmother a thousand times: "Just look at little Suzy, how beautifully she plays the piano." "Just look at little Suzy, who speaks English perfectly!" Suzy was a distant family member whom I hated with all my heart. I didn't even know her; we never met until we became fellow students at university. And we became good friends and have stayed friends ever since.

I hated to be compared to her. I was incredibly angry that somebody was put in front of me as a measure, someone who was always a level higher than me no matter what I did. With all the "look-at-her," I wasn't given an achievable goal or encouraging support, but I felt downgraded.

My children have the "look-at-little-Suzy" comments to thank that it doesn't even occur to me to compare them to anyone else, be they an acquaintance, a classmate, or a sibling. In our house, there's no "See how well the other has finished their food!" or "Most of your classmates could learn it, so how come you couldn't?" or "Tidy up your desk to make it look as nice as your brother's!" That wouldn't achieve anything apart from creating tension. Whoever is ranked lower by my comparison would be angry with the other one who is labelled better than them. They'd grow jealous of them as well as angry with me. It'd also be a suicide attempt as I'd encourage them to compete by comparing, when what actually gets on my nerves the most is the recurrent competition between them when they want to put down/outdo each other, anyway.

If I insist on making comparisons, I should compare him to himself. "Last time you tidied up your writing cabinet so nicely, could you do it like that again?" If I put it like this, I'm also saying to him that the possibility is in you, you just have to find it and I trust that you'll be able to do so. However, I need to proceed carefully in this field, too. When I introduce the "look at" tone against himself, like "look at how nice you were when you were small," that's not about giving acceptance, trust, support and encouragement; it's more like holding him accountable for his current self and placing an expectation on him to change.

The "just look at" is a mixture of degradation and encouragement: you're not as good as him but I'd like you to be, I hope that you can achieve the same. If I take out the former and just express encouragement – go on, be brave, you can do it, come on, trust yourself, go for it! – I can inspire far more effectively.

Wisdom for the road:

"All good things must come to an end."

"Life is not a bowl of cherries."

"All beginnings are difficult."

"Everything has a price."

"Washing dishes is woman's work."

Words of wisdom such as these were passed on to me by books and different family members, words I could travel through life with. And they added "Like it or not, that's what you're getting!" So, I've been nibbling on these snacks for years. Then I realised there's such a variety of different snacks available: apples on the tree, bread in the supermarket, cakes made by our neighbours. I love the snacks I've been given, but it's great that there are so many different things I can choose from!

Remembering

I remember my mother sitting next to my bed every single night while I was falling asleep. I put myself down for years for not being as good a mother; I run out of energy by the evening and I don't feel like sitting next to anybody. I told my mother about this not so long ago and it turns out that she puts herself down to this day for not sitting next to me enough.

Picture this: One of my sons falls on concrete from a height, loses consciousness, and has to be taken to hospital in an ambulance. He keeps saying: "Mama, don't leave me alone." I won't. I keep talking to him. I keep my hand on him, so he can feel that I'm with him in every way possible. I don't let him be pushed into the room while I'm giving his details on the ward. I don't even go to the toilet until a relative takes my place at his side. It's only the X-ray where I'm not allowed to go with him. I sleep next to him on the floor, putting my hand on his bed, holding his hand all night. And what does he remember the following day? Nothing. Except that he was on his own in the X-ray.

So be careful with those memories, because what the child remembers and how they remember events cannot always be influenced either by the parent or by the facts themselves.

4

From the ideal age difference to sibling training

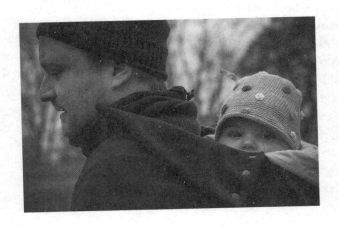

I think children are like amoebas: they fill all available space no matter how many of them there are. I've been a mother of one, but I don't believe that life with one is any easier than life with two or three or even more. Difficulties on the physical level may be in direct proportion to the number of children, as three beings usually eat three times more than one. And if they're of different ages and personalities, which is highly likely to be the case with any number of children, there are more demands which require a larger infrastructure.

However, I often see that raising one child comes with questions that may make everyday life harder than having more children. What will happen to the child once the parent is gone? Should they have a sibling or not? Should the child carry on the family's music or sporting lineage? Do parents need to be constantly available when the child requires a playmate? When the attention is divided between more children, parents usually get off lightly with there not being too much attention needed for every single one. When one child is my everything, I can be lost in being a mother the same way as when I'm buried under the tasks of being a parent of several kids. Most areas of difficulty are the same, no matter the number of children; however, there are a number of things that, by the nature of them, are voiced only by parents of two or more. For example, how to give everyone an equal amount of risotto, time, or attention.

Ideal age difference

Sometimes I feel that there are people who are not as into having another child as much as finding the ideal age difference. There should be a year between them, so that they grow close quickly, so that they can entertain each other and we get over the hard bit in one go. The older one should be three (four with Waldorf parents) when the next one comes along, so that they go to nursery school and I can be at home with just the little one during the day. Let the age difference be even bigger, so that the first born can help with the younger one.

I have children born twenty minutes and eleven years apart. The former is like studying at two or three universities at the same time; I have a few minutes a week to think about me existing as a separate entity, other than to satisfy the needs and wishes of the children, even though I mostly enjoy the job. Of course, it must be easier to do this with more help – a live-in granny, or not breastfeeding at night or at all – but I'm not familiar with such options. However, when the age difference is small, there's much connection, with many common experiences; there's a childhood spent together.

And when the children are older, there's a witness to what they've lived through when they were little. As a mother, it's fantastic to watch as the defensive and offensive alliance is formed day by day between siblings with a small age difference. When the younger child is around, those "let's join forces" looks become more common between siblings, and interactions, giving and taking, exchanging and bargaining, become daily occurrences. There are big laughs together rolling on the floor like lion cubs on the mattress, as they pull, drag, and bite one another. They learn how far the other

91

extends, what hurts, what causes the other pain. They also use each other as mirrors: I'm not as small as you; I'm a boy, you're a girl; I like being tickled more than you. A non-stop course in self-image. It's good to watch as they giggle, as they close in, as they join their strengths – I can enjoy this even when it happens to be directed against me. Within reason, of course.

If I give birth when the bigger one is in preschool or the age difference is even greater, I may live in the hope that the older one will sit down and play with the shape sorter and the little one. But I quickly realise that he is far more interested in the shape and form of the opposite sex. There's also the advantage that the teenager does not scratch the young one's eyes out when his ball is taken. Moreover, the little one has the choice not only of following parental behavioural patterns, but also of copying their older siblings, while the older one may let his heart melt freely by the sweetness of the little one, perhaps tinted with fewer or easier-to-handle feelings of jealousy. The way the older one teaches the one a metre shorter than him to walk, the way he protects him at the playground from an attack by his playmates and from falling off the slide, the way he sits him on his lap and tells him a story – it melts my heart instantly, just seeing in their looks and their movements how much they adore each other.

Well, these are the things that make being a mother worthwhile. No one age difference is ideal and at the same time they all are, if I can see them that way.

Daily doses

"How do you make fifteen minutes a day for every one of your children?" my friend asks. I don't. Definitely not every day and it's not my goal either. The reason being that I consider the forming of a good basic relationship more important and that's supported by two major pillars: on the one hand I should notice which one of my children needs me that day, and on the other hand I'm able to be the sort of mother (I have that kind of connection with them) who they feel comfortable asking for, or even demanding, attention, should they require it of me.

I don't want to push myself down their throats. Sometimes they don't even need me for fifteen minutes a day. And if they do need me, they don't always need fifteen minutes. I can see that he's sad, I take him aside and give him a hug without a word – it can be worth as much as thirty-five minutes of attention.

Touch is not required to the same extent by every child either. I have a child who has loved physical contact from birth and still feels happiest when tied to me. No, I'm not talking about the twelve-year-old. I've also got a child who only liked cuddling at bedtime. Do I stroke and kiss all my children every morning when they go off? There are ones who like being kissed less and my ten-year-old reacts to stroking by biting my head off with more passion than a hungry lion. Well, I had messed up his carefully set hairstyle, one he'd spent so much time on. He's right, I wasn't paying attention to his wishes. I can still stroke his head at bedtime when it no longer matters that I flatten his hair.

And there's also the question of for whom, for what, to what extent, and in what form I have a need. Well, that's a multitude of layers and segments – what a lot of possibilities!

Children's room

Imagine this scenario: there are five kids in the children's room, three of whom are testosterone bombs running around with eardrum-ripping battle cries. They're shooting, throwing themselves on the floor, jumping, buzzing. I'd be happy to peacefully engage in some baby play in the middle of the room either with my own youngest or with my daughter's dolls, but it bothers me, more and more by the second, that they're running around me screaming. I hate that there is no peace.

"Mama, what's the matter?" one of the warriors stops over me, as he sees my face distorting.

"You're so loud!" I tell him, puffing.

"Well, this is the children's room and you're sitting in the middle of it, where, by the way, you're in the way, and you're not willing to be running around with weapons either, so if you can't be louder and more active, then there is the adult room!"

OMG, another baby

When I found out that I had conceived my fifth child, I wept. I was petrified that I wouldn't survive it, that I wouldn't be strong enough to cope when things got even harder than they already were. I often detect in myself that when I think of change, I imagine that everything stays exactly the same as it is at present, with an extra layer added on top. The days will be the same except there will be someone else there to bring additional tasks by their mere existence.

The nature of change, however, is not like this at all. It's more like when I add a new colour to a wet watercolour painting. The new colour changes the existing colours, the original lines move, the texture of the paper changes. In fact, the child doesn't even have to be born for the changes that take place in me during my pregnancy to occur, changes which can result in shifts visible in everyday life. It's also possible that I get to the stage when I sprinkle my days with more help and so the birth of a new child actually makes everyday life easier than before.

Me, the control freak

What can lie behind the phenomenon that it often makes me feel secure to have control? For example, horrendous fear.

Living the life of a mother of five children means that I could be an Olympic medallist in logistics. Lunch is usually ready by 9am so that we can go and discover the world with the smaller children in the morning. Then we have to get home by midday for lunch and afternoon sleep protocols to follow dutifully by 1pm. A table laid with lunch must be waiting for the bigger children returning from school. Should the simultaneous afternoon sleep of the two small ones not happen in the time period, the next question is whether the youngest one should be allowed to fall asleep at 3pm or later in the car on the way to the older sibling's training. But if we go to training, who will be in for the guitar teacher? Should I lay the table for dinner before we leave, because by the time we get home, everyone will be exhausted and sometimes whether we can all eat together is down to those two-minute tasks, like laying the table. Should the little ones have a bath after dinner or should it be story time first, or should I hang out the washing instead? And there's that meat for tomorrow's lunch I mustn't forget to take out of the freezer.

What happens if I let go of all control and just allow things to happen as they do? That's scary, as I've experienced it before. If there's no lunch, if we skip it or it's just late, whether there's sleep time or no sleep time, whether we get home or don't get home on time, when I don't sign stuff, forget to take things out, don't prepare in advance... Mountains of frustration. Although it's not easy to keep control either, leaving myself to the mercy of the uncontrollable is definitely the harder bite for me. Routine is like a fence: I can lean on it, it contains things. At the same time, it keeps me in a realm and doesn't let me step outside to see the world the way I would sometimes like to. The monotonous repetition of routine devours my brain after a while if I don't pay attention and make small changes every day, new motions, undiscovered colours and tastes.

My friend, who is also a mother of five, lives life with considerably less routine, in a more relaxed manner. There's not so much consistency in their daily life as there is in ours. I admire her. And she admires me.

Recharging

It's one thing that the big one looks after the small one sometimes – even if he pulls a face about it – and that I don't need to help all my children to put their shoes on any more. But I also have more important, deeper experiences about the advantages of a big age difference. When I was thirteen, my brother was born, at fifteen my sister. Playing mummy with them felt so good. At that time, I was often uncomfortable in my own skin. Neither school nor home was great. They were like an island for the shipwrecked where instead of cold winds, the sun shone warmly. There was firm ground under my feet, so my stomach stopped churning from the sea tossing me about and there were always coconuts on the palm tree. They were my recharging places. The love that I could give to just a few people at the time could be given to them without inhibition and it was equally easy for me to accept love from them.

Now that I've also managed to produce the large age difference, further aspects get to shine. I can see that for me, as their mother, being with one is helped by the existence of the other. When the young ones take all my strength with the night and day shifts – bedtime, feeding, cooking, repeating rhymes, playground trips twice a day, whatdoesthedonkeysay? heehaw – then it's ever so refreshing to discuss meaningful stuff in grown-up language with the big kids, or to play a board game with them or read *The Lord of the Rings* instead of *Paddington Bear*. Conversely, when it's a bumpier ride with the big children, when they're pushing the boundaries or each other, I can draw considerably from putting my focus on one of the smaller children cuddling up to me, or I tie them to me and just keep singing, singing, singing to them without a thought in my head.

What are siblings for?

I've never been an only child and as a mother of twins, I've never had one child. However, I do have five children from two relationships and I have all kinds of siblings, full, half, and step included. There are ones I've grown up with and ones I've never lived with. My connection to each of them is very different.

With my brother, there's a kind of connection I don't share with anyone else. We have the same mother, the same father, the same childhood. With him being the older one, he also guards many of my early memories – it's funny and interesting that sometimes his recollection is totally different from mine. I can use this to put a different light on things. If I move a lamp in a dark room to a new place, I will see different things or a different side to things. We can remember the same event with totally different emotional content. Apart from this being funny, it also accurately shows that there's no such thing as something being good or bad, or our parental patterns being good or bad, but I instinctively code events and place them in my useful and not useful boxes. And what else does this mean? It also means that I can re-label them, too.

The good thing about siblings is that they keep. In our adolescence, my older brother and I had a year when we were really close, with many deep conversations. I was very close to my younger sister and brother in their younger years. I'm in daily contact with one of my siblings, even though she doesn't even live in this country. Siblings don't disappear from your life. If you have many of them, it's great that you can connect closely with different ones at different times.

When my brother was busy chasing girls, I was often busy grieving for the loss of my daily connection with him. For a long time, I wanted to get back the brother I used to spend my time with, talk to, argue with, the one who would hit me, the one who would pay attention to me in whatever way. Our once so close and good relationship did not return for a long while. For this I blamed him, myself, and fate interchangeably. Then one day I realised that if this was so important to me I could do something for the relationship instead of whining about it. We already had fairly big children of our own when

I approached him to tell him that I missed him and that we should spend more time together. I arranged for the four children to be looked after at home. He was also a busy, hard-working father, but we still managed to make time for a weekly chat. It was good to get back to being siblings and experience the great richness of having a big brother again.

I've gained and still get much from not having had a break from children. When I was growing out of my childhood, my younger brother was born, then two years later, my younger sister, and as they were growing up – my little brother was twelve, my sister ten – my first children were born. This way I don't feel and have never felt the "young people these days" sentiment. I don't feel a generation gap. Instead, I feel transition, familiarity, so I can easily and quickly access my child and the young adult self in me.

And yes, my siblings and me are there for each other in times of need, not even just a little. When our mother was in prison, we closed together airtight; we held and completed one another; we formed a circle, a globe, a sheath. It was an incredible help that there were people around me who did not ask how I was feeling, they just felt it themselves.

Wishing is an art form

During my first pregnancy, I decided that I didn't want to know whether I was going to have a boy or a girl. "So, what do you feel you're having?" I was asked every hour. "Well, if I really focus inward and listen to my tiny inner voice," I said, "I feel it's a girl." This girl ended up being two boys... so much for mother's insight!

The second time, I secretly trusted that I would have a girl but inwardly and outwardly I said that the gender was all the same to me, the main thing was that the baby was healthy. For I couldn't even admit to myself that I wanted a girl. I grew up in a family with a social pattern according to which I have to accept what I get and be happy about what I'm given. I interpreted this as if I wished for a girl and I had a boy, then I'd have committed a sin of some sort. Furthermore, I was able to support this theory with data: I reread in my university notes that it had been empirically proven that if one wishes strongly for a child of a certain gender and then the baby turns out to be of the opposite sex, it's far more likely that the child will suffer from an identity crisis in later life – so I might even harm my child with my desires.

Expecting my fourth child, my husband longed to know the gender of our baby in advance. I was mulling over it relentlessly, I was trying to push my thoughts about whatever will be will be great down my own throat. Let's enjoy the excitement of the expectancy, we'll have plenty of time to be looking at the sexual organs for years after the birth. Then one day, I took a deep breath and went to see my sonographer on my own. I asked him to write the sex of the baby on the picture without telling me and place it in an envelope. The following night I gave my husband this envelope for our anniversary.

He opened the envelope and wow, a girl! And there, in a split second, I realised how much I had been longing for a girl and what enormous amounts of strength I had mobilised to deny this even to myself. With my barriers collapsed, my expectations of myself dissolved into thin air.

My most prominent feeling, however, was not one of joy. It felt really scary. I was confused. To breastfeed a girl? Ooooh, how do you do that? To give birth to a baby girl, to change her nappy?! I'm already good at vrooming, sword fighting and playing football, but what am I going to do with pink ponies? On reflection my questions seem ridiculous, but they gnawed at me then, despite not being a first-time mother, but having had three children already. Facing suppressed desires and entering an unknown territory can be terribly frightening.

Why is having a daughter as well so good?

Having a daughter in addition to my sons is good. It's good because it won't be at the crucial moment that my son sees a fanny for the first time.

Fair

Is it fair if I divide the chocolate or the risotto unevenly? It is one of my kids' favourite, the others like it, and one isn't that keen on it. If I dish out the same amount for everyone, that seems fair. But why should the one who doesn't like it so much or feel like having it, have to eat the same amount or any of it at all? Why shouldn't the one whose favourite food it is have some extra? Am I being fair when all my children get exactly the same attention? Am I being fair if I spend fifteen minutes a day with each one of them? If one of them wants to do nothing that afternoon apart from reading *Winnetou*, should I still drag them away from their book because I've already spent time with my other children that day, reading to them and playing with them, so should I force my attention on this child? Is it fair if I ask my children who come home from school early to hang out the washing three times a week or should I hand out the task evenly, making the one who gets home just in time for dinner do the same amount as the others? Am I being fair when I enjoy being with one of them more that particular day because it's easier to spend time together, while my relationship is less easy at that time with the other? Am I being a good mother if I don't give all my children the same amount, the same way, at the same time?

Mentally it's easy for me to understand that responding according to need (including my own needs) means something different with all my children. To make this knowledge even deeper, to believe in it to the core, to not question myself but let myself act automatically according to their various needs, is sometimes not such a smooth ride for me. When I get stuck, I'll re-read these few lines. And if that still doesn't work, then instead of guilt – that I've done everything wrong and I cannot change it ever again – I will try to trust at least that I've made the same mistakes, doing things wrong to all my children equally.

Oppressor or victim?
Or just sibling training

A friend of mine feels sorry for her daughter because she's constantly being picked on by her brother. My acquaintances sometimes pity my third son for being oppressed by his brothers, for being picked on and teased. There was a time when I could really feel sorry for myself for my brother hitting me, picking on me, teasing me. Although I was not vocal about it, even as a small child I was aware of how I also had a good part to play in those situations. To this day I can remember that at around the age of four or five I would annoy my brother and then when he finally pushed me, I'd call for an adult, wailing, begging for him to be told off. I'd cry theatrically while being sardonically happy inside that my plan had paid off. Even back then I knew – or rather sensed – exactly how he worked and how adults worked. I could take advantage of the cracks in their shields as the workings of those living with me were rather predictable.

And this is not even the really important part today. The important thing is how much good there was for me in my brother being such a tease and a wind-up merchant. I learnt from it. Many, many parts of me have been formed thanks to this. Having experienced it myself, I knew for sure that my brother was strong – and later on, when he used his strength to protect me, he made me feel very safe. Sibling training actually made me physically strong as well, just like play-fighting does for lion cubs. I was never afraid to go home in the dark. However, I never wanted to be like him, I never wanted to fight, to struggle, to show off my strength the way he'd done. I didn't feel oppressed, it felt really good to be different; him being one way helped me define myself in another. Indeed, I was able to use my seemingly oppressed status to make people feel sorry for me, but when I look deep inside myself, it wasn't so tragic.

Which doesn't mean that I watch idly when any of my children physically or verbally hurt any one of the others. I keep talking in vain, fighting a losing battle while I know that probably one day, inexorably and unstoppably, it'll all sort itself out and we'll get past this phase. One day, they'll stop fighting one another as the outside world, friends, and girls become more exciting; picking on one another will no longer appeal quite so much.

Boundaries

In our house, you're not allowed to eat outside the kitchen. "May I eat in my room? Just this once... I'll take a plate in. Then I'll bring it out. I'd love to have some tea in my bed while I'm reading."

In our house, you're not allowed to go inside with your shoes on. "May I go in? Just for a jumper, please; if I take my shoes off I'll be late! We're leaving in ten minutes anyway, please don't make me take my shoes off till then, ok, just this once, all right?"

In our house, there's no watching movies during the week. "May I watch a video? Please, it's only three minutes, really! May I check who won the match yesterday? Can we watch a twenty-minute cartoon in the evening, you know, that sweet one!"

In our house, you're not allowed to get up from the dinner table until everyone is finished. "May I go to my room? My homework is not done yet. May I leave the table? I am so tired... I'm so full, I must lie down!"

In our house boundaries are only good for wiping our bums with – but if we didn't have them, what would we wipe our bums with?

Experience doesn't help

With every single birth I grew more and more afraid of what was ahead of me/us. It became clearer that I couldn't get used to this pain, I couldn't predict the blocks or sort out all physical-emotional problems mentally in advance. Perhaps it's true here as well that blessed are the poor in spirit – at least it was ignorance and lack of experience that helped me expect my first child in a cloud-free state. Oh, giving birth hurts so much that some all but die from it? Well, I won't, mine won't hurt so much, I can take it! I'll get through it with a straight spine. Hmmm … I didn't think any of this later.

Getting to the terrible twos, my stomach began to tighten at smaller and smaller tantrums thinking 'ohmygodwhatistherestilltocome.' The fear in me grew more and more about things getting tougher and I feared that I wouldn't survive this one easily, as I hadn't got through the previous ones lightly either. Not without struggle, surely – which I wasn't any more into, just because I'd gained experience of it. With the first children, I believed in myself and I enthusiastically repeated a mantra that it didn't matter, although the tantrum was approaching, I would stay in control, make it through, come to a solution, even if standing on one leg, no matter what. Hmmm... now I'm already dreading the tantrums of the fifth child even though the fourth one is just starting them.

When experience plants fear in me, it obstructs the free flow of things and limits my actions. If I make myself aware of this, I can figure out that I'm petrified now because of my previous birth experiences. If I realise that it's not because of the current tantrum that my stomach knots but rather the result of past tantrums, then I free some blocked parts of me and I can become operational again.

Experience helps

At the time my first children were born I thought that the purpose of the puerperium* is that all relatives and

---

* The period of about six weeks after childbirth during which the mother's reproductive organs return to their original non-pregnant condition.

acquaintances could come and visit, to admire the child. They could bring some non-slip socks for them and some cream cakes for me. Well, that was dreadful. It took a week for the first round of visits to be over and just like at a Picasso exhibition, there was a queue. Then they made contact a week later saying that they wanted to visit again. Three or four visits a day, everyone staying an hour to an hour and a half, then we washed up the cups and plates for the next lot. I didn't even notice how tired I got from all the smiling, from not giving myself time to listen inward, to get to know my babies, to get on the same wavelength, to rest through the contractions of my uterus. I was ashamed that my clothes were stained with breastmilk. I'd leave the room to breastfeed feeling embarrassed. I should've politely said that the visits were no longer pleasant, that I couldn't rest and be with my babies. I'd just given birth and in truth, I should have only been doing the latter two things with short intervals, not entertaining a stream of visitors.

Next time, I will say in advance: please stay for only ten to fifteen minutes. Before you come, ask my husband what you should bring. Look at the sweet little baby, share our joy briefly and then leave, taking the rubbish down to the collection point with you. Oh, and please don't use strong scents because it's a cruel blow when that wonderfully delicate baby smell is exterminated by perfume.

The first puerperium showed me how important it is to pay attention to myself and my own needs. I've learnt to guard and keep the irreplaceable, unique softness and intimacy of those first few days after the birth for my baby, for myself and my newborn family.

Hormones

Children in their terrible twos, adolescents, and expectant mothers are equally defenceless and thrown about by hormones. There's no consistency. Predictability is rare, but suddenly there are tons of unexpected reactions with astoundingly high amplitude to all sorts of phenomena. It's hard to live with them all, and whichever life phase you're in, it's also hard to live with oneself. If I'm lucky, I'll get off lightly by not having to accommodate all three life phases at the same time in my family.

Translation engine

The number of children I have equals the number of languages I speak. Each one has a different favourite dish, each one is ticklish in a different spot, each one can be reached in a different way if I want to hear about their joy or sadness. When one of them asks what there is for dinner, I know he's very hungry. When the other one asks, I know he's worried it'll be something he doesn't like that much. When it comes to the third one, I know that he's not hungry, and when it's the fourth, I know that she'd like to be offended that, yet again, it's not what she has requested so many times (and we just had it two days before). I know from the tones of their voices, their body language. I know from the emotional state they've been in lately. I know how their bodies work. I know when they last had something to eat and around about what time they will get hungry again. I like about me that I know them, that I can guess their thoughts. I like that our connection is so deep, that there are so many strings tied together, that I can see them and their feelings without words or see their desires beyond their words.

And this vast knowledge also has its limitations. I notice that at times I react according to my assumptions. When I perceive a question as my daughter looking for an opportunity to get offended, I take it as an attack and there's either defensiveness or tension in my response, so we get into a sort of game.

I don't like playing such games, so I try to change this. I become a translating machine. I simultaneously interpret in four directions: to me about me, to me about them, to them about me, and to them about them. Instead of my perceptions, I ask questions. In the first round, I examine myself – I try to do something against being the banana skin on which our clear communication slips. Is it certain that whatever I'm thinking is what's actually going on in my child? Then I ask him: "Are you sure this is what you wanted to ask? Because for some reason I feel that your question has a different meaning." At this time, it often turns out that I've wrongly assumed, and he'd asked exactly what he had wanted to ask. Or it turns out that it was indeed not what he had wanted to find out but something completely different, something that I'd never have suspected. Or it turns out that I was right and, from then on, we communicate clearly about what the real content is. I make my inner thoughts transparent to him, even the assumptions I've made about him. From there we can move on to a different dimension, further and further in, gradually towards the more significant stuff. It's so beautiful that even a simple "What's for dinner" is so vividly complex.

Silence police

One of the hardest things for me in having many children is that silence is rare, yet there's plenty of demand for it. I guard the sleep of my bigger children against my one-year-old who wakes up at 5am and is totally unwilling to understand the meaning of shush, laughing aloud instead. We simply spend the next two or three hours in our seven-square-meter kitchen – I take him on a journey through the world of fridge magnets, we cook lunch, and he eats half the fridge by the time the sun comes up. When we've exhausted all the kitchen has to offer, we rearrange the shoes in the hall or like two angels we have the evening bath over and done with at 6am. By the time the slightly older one wakes up, the youngest is feeling sleepy so from then on, we should be careful not to wake him up. After lunch, it's nap time for the small ones and quiet time for the big ones, for a change. Then, after a few hours' break, the evening comes, and the two sections of the children's room fall asleep with as much as an hour and half's difference. I hate constantly telling someone to be quieter. When I want to sneak out, I hate waiting on tiptoes for the bus to pass under the window so that it will drown out the noise of the creaking floor, which is loud enough to wake those half-asleep. All my bits hate being a silence-chief. I hate that I can't find a way out of this so that the problem disappears from our lives for good. Only momentarily, only sometimes am I capable of being creative enough not to feel bad. I'm looking forward so much to nobody sleeping during the day, which means I'm really looking forward to being two years on from now, just like I used to look forward to my birthdays when I was little. Of course, there are times when I step out of the routine, go for a walk at 5am; there are times when I don't put them down in the day because I feel that I'll find it easier to cope with the dead-tired child later; there are times when I let everyone be noisy and sometimes I even reach the point when I don't mind one waking up the other because what will be will be. However, I haven't managed to find a real, long-standing solution as yet; policing for silence has not disappeared from my life. I've noticed that lately I've become envious of larger apartments because our small living space aggravates the problem. Please give me a bigger home or some useful advice.

Argue-machines

I keep telling the two-and-a-half-year-old that it's possible to talk to the one-year-old. She should make him understand, explain to him what she's doing and why, ask for the toy she wants and reason with him for an exchange. I teach the five-year-old about techniques of persuasion so that he's adequately equipped to convince his brother to choose the cartoon he also wants to watch.

Then, when they figure that they'd like to have a cat and gang up on me to argue for it, well that feels like holding my own machine gun, dutifully cleaned twice a day, looking into the barrel, and pulling the trigger.

Survival mode

Yes, there is such a thing. I've been in survival mode for years. Raising three children alone was very often a struggle for survival. Like, let me just survive this day. When at 7am

I'm looking forward to 8pm as if waiting for the Messiah. When success is that the day was not as unsuccessful as the one before. When I see it as good that on that day I only shouted once and not all evening. When the unexpected things hit me in the stomach, for example, please don't let me or them be ill because there's no reserve. When I'm dreading the summer break as if I had to get through a dark forest in the middle of the night with black knights on my tail. And thinking all the time that I'm doing something wrong; I keep lashing myself with an imaginary whip.

And then, when years later my friend is in the same boat, I'm able to look at her situation and through this, at my former self. I didn't actually do that badly. This is the nature of the genre. There are such periods, months, days, hours. Of course, it must be possible to get through these in a thousand different ways, but I often didn't manage to find any other way. I can tell my friend now what I couldn't tell myself then: you're doing incredibly well, your daily life is working! The small invisible cogwheels are turning; the kids don't go hungry – there's food on the table every day, even if it's just frankfurters; they're not in after-school club every day till half past five; they're not sitting in front of the TV for two hours a day; there's enough energy left to show them the world; they're given story time, hugs, kisses, and care every day; they go training; they learn poems together for school; they can invite their friends around; there's lots of laughing together and I could go on. I didn't realise that even in survival mode they got so much good from me!

The joys of having many children

There's constant movement in the house, there's continuous chirping. Three pounds of meat and four pounds of potatoes are eaten in seven minutes. We fill the No.16 bus. I have to think of forty presents for the eight days of Hanukkah. I'm always needed. I can play with Duplo as early as 6am. There's no family ticket which includes us all without a supplement. It's story time several times a day; I hear the voice of cartoon characters more than my husband's. I get to eat all the apple peel and bread crust.

The difficulties of having many children

There's constant movement in the house, there's continuous chirping. Three pounds of meat and four pounds of potatoes are eaten in seven minutes. We fill the No.16 bus. I have to think of forty presents for the eight days of Hanukkah. I'm always needed. I can play with Duplo as early as 6am. There's no family ticket which includes us all without a supplement. It's story time several times a day; I hear the voice of cartoon characters more than my husband's. I get to eat all the apple peel and bread crust.

5

Instead of giving advice on how to raise children

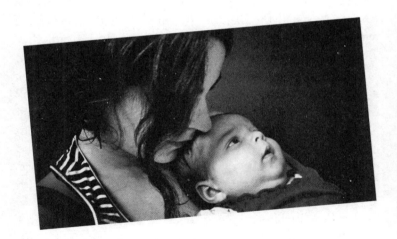

It's hard to find a good word that describes living with children. *Education* refers to a deliberate, purposeful act, although I do things both consciously and unconsciously when I'm with my kids. *Upbringing* and *raising* children suggest to me that the kids would grow up without me anyway, so I like to use *parenting* to describe the way I like to be when I'm a mother.

Children learn from what I tell them, but also from observing my concrete actions and what's behind them; they pick up how to use mascara, or how to be a woman. My children understand from my unconscious movements and my gestures if we're afraid of dogs. Even when we're not with our children, we still provide them with a pattern by the way we exist in the world. They internalise whether we fight to realise our dreams or give up on them. They see when we choose to spend the majority of our time with them and if we don't, they see what it is we choose to do instead. They don't learn from us the way they learn at school – even if that would be ever so much simpler! Today's lesson, my children, is on how to be unselfish with your siblings. Open the book on page twenty-five. I can raise my children to be unselfish directly, with my words, but if they hear me on the phone to my brother the following day apologetically refusing to lend him my car as I'm worried about the damage he might cause, I instantly wipe out the values I was trying to pass on with my words.

I believe in genuine living together. This does not mean I must be a saint. In fact, if my children consider me to be one, they'll probably be really struggling with their self-esteem. What it means is congruence, what is inside is out and vice versa. I have the courage to show my value system, my successes, my shameful decisions, my joys, my sadness. I don't have to put everything on display; that's not what will make me true in their eyes. However, whatever I do display and whatever I choose not to show, even though they can sense it – as children feel the invisible as well as hear the unsaid – is round and complete. No matter how much I'm aware of this and believe in it, living this way requires continuous introspection. Unconsciously, it has an effect on the level of my actions, and if there's a contradiction between the two, some dirt enters the working machinery. My child senses the lack of congruence and becomes uncertain, or I become inauthentic in their eyes. So, to put it simply, childrearing, or genuine living together, is self-knowledge and self-acceptance itself.

This book does not aim to give advice on raising children. I describe situations, and share thoughts that can be inspiring. There are a few tips included, but if anyone feels they're not for them, as they have a different temperament or value system, they'll not opt for using them anyway – and that qualifies neither my ideas, nor the person who chooses to ignore them. And at other times, it's precisely an idea that is directly opposite our views that can help us move forward or nudge us out of a difficult position.

Abandonment

There are very few things I swore to do before I had children and out of those few, probably the only one I stand by to this day is never to say to my child "I'll leave you here if you don't come now." I don't ever say this because I know how the message insidiously seeps in as he gradually becomes terrified. I know how strongly his anxiety and fear can stop him from feeling safe with me.

When one of my kids was seven, he climbed a tree in anger while the rest of us played football a few metres away, letting him act offended. After two goals, I looked up; he wasn't there. Uh-oh, my stomach instantly shrank to the size of a cherry pit and I began to sweat, worry, shiver, and despair.

A few minutes later he appeared. My heart tightened as I imagined what he must have been going through and I asked, with my voice breaking as I was close to tears, whether he'd been feeling scared thinking that we'd left him. And he replied: "But Mama, why would I have been scared? You would never leave here without me!"

And there and then I felt as deeply as never before how the little things we do every day really do add up to a lot.

They don't read

The oldest kids are in fifth grade but I'm really bothered by the fact that they don't read regularly. Of course, I know that basically I'm also longing for some peaceful time, relaxing in bed so that I can immerse myself in a book. But this is not only a projection of my own desire, it would also be lovely to see them sucked in by a piece of writing, simply for the fact that reading is a unique source of joy, a well of pleasure irreplaceable by any other.

I'm trying to read more and more interesting books to them, trying to find what their contemporaries like. I have a system: we allocate time for reading together in case routine whets the appetite. I try to ask nicely. I attempt to make it compulsory. All to no avail.

Fine, then. We need another way. Prohibiting and rewarding comes to mind. I can't think of any form of prohibition I believe in. Rewarding has more chance, but one bar of chocolate for each book seems silly. What is it that they really want, and can I relate it to reading somehow? And the idea pops up: that's it, to stay awake for longer! There's not a single bedtime they're not begging for more, just ten more minutes, pleeease. Well, then, all right, if you're reading in bed, you can stay up an extra half hour; if you're not, it's time to sleep. Since that day I can safely say they love reading.

Childish

"Stop being so childish!" says a mother to her nineteen-month-old baby who gets bored after sitting pretty for ten minutes.

When the child is a few days old, we're looking forward to getting a smile back. When they're a few weeks old, we're looking forward to our baby turning, then crawling. When they're six months old, we're looking forward to them standing up. When they're a year old, it would be great if they started walking and talking as well. At two, it's time for potty training or else they won't be admitted to nursery at the age of three. When they have to be carried a lot, we're looking forward to them walking and getting further away from us and then we complain that they hardly ever climb into our lap any more. It's not all right when their bags have to be carried for them to school, but then we're not happy either when they carry all their stuff themselves and go off ahead because they're embarrassed to be seen with us.

To enjoy the present, the here and now, is a great little task; to get high on the moment's happiness, to be amazed by what they can do today, is very important because whatever they do today, they'll not do it again the same way tomorrow. I take a long deep breath to slow my brain down from rushing ahead, to focus my attention, to allow those plentiful small details, stick in my mind. This is great for me as those little, frozen moments will become my memories. And this is great for the child, too, as they can fully live in their present and can then progress to the next phase, free of trauma, with natural ease.

Saying no

Why is it good for my children that I don't allow everything? If I let them do anything, how would they develop? Would they learn to fight for a better life? I don't know. All I know for sure is that when I put up a wall, and it's made of rubber, lined with love, then they don't get hurt when they bump into it and even if they do, they don't suffer permanent damage. Just as my body grew throughout the course of my pregnancies, my boundaries have taken new shape all the time, daily, ever since. I'm not being consistent by rigidly sticking to my principles, just as a baby couldn't healthily grow inside me, if my body were not to change its shape. Equally, it's also unimaginable to be without any boundaries at all, else why the embracing uterus or the protecting amniotic sac? Would it be good for the children in tsunamis of hysterics and teenage hormonal volcanic eruptions if they were left flowing boundlessly? Would that serve them well in the short or long term? I believe that I do right by being their wall sometimes because by doing so, I protect them and contain them, and in the meantime, I slowly and gradually let them out, let them through and let them go.

Sweets police

I don't always like my policing role. To guard their sleep, to make sure they eat healthy, to decide whether they're allowed to jump off from a height of two metres, to set boundaries 147 times a day. Much of this happens routinely and so it doesn't bother me too much. Many instances I can look at as interesting questions, but there are returning elements that drive me up the wall.

There was a rule for my kids, for example, that they shouldn't eat sweets all the time; they could have one after school lunch and after dinner. With boundaries comes the testing of boundaries: "Please, Mama, just one more. Just a little, just a bit, pleeeease." I hated it. They would look at me with their big, sad, doggy eyes and I'd say no as my head said no but my heart is soft as butter, of course. And naturally, they could sense that, and they'd launch their offensive and drop their bombs and I'd have to withstand the attack. Naaah. One day I got fed up and played with the thought: what would happen if they could eat as much as they wanted to? This was a little scary for me as with five children, on the one hand, this could mean that the drawer would be emptied within two days after shopping, and on the other, I was afraid that they'd eat way too much unhealthy sugary stuff. I was, however, so very fed up with my 'policewoman of sweets' role that I was happy to pass the uniform on to them. "You know that it's unhealthy to eat too much sweet stuff. You know that each person works differently every day – some days I'd like more, some days none at all – and you also know that we shop once a week; so, put these three things together and eat as much as you like." I give the control over to them and I watch the unfolding events with interest.

They become trainee policemen. They have to control themselves and each other. Sometimes they still asked, "Are we allowed three sweets today?" and many times they proudly reported "I've only had one today." The sweets drawer is not emptied in two days; stocks sometimes last even longer than in the past. They claim that they prefer to control the sweets themselves – and I definitely enjoy having been able to hang up my uniform. The new system is working.

After a few weeks one of the kids cuddles up and says: "It was a little bit better when you told us how much we could have…" "Why?" I ask in surprise. "Because you always allowed us to have a little bit more, but I never allow myself." Well, yes, an FBI agent is ruthless with himself, too.

Instead of labelling

We set off to climb the steps to the castle (all 179 of them) and she's tired. As soon as she looks at the distance ahead, she asks to be picked up. Her younger brother is on my back, the plastic motorbike in my hand, but I can take it. Of course I can; I'm strong. Halfway, nearly at the point of collapse, I tell her that the moment has come for me to put her down. "Why? she asks. "Because you're heavy," I label routinely. "I'm not heavy!" she protests passionately, screaming, upset, raging. She stalls, refuses to go on. "You know what, you're completely right! You're not heavy. The thing is that I cannot carry you, or rather I cannot carry all the things I have on me. Your brother cannot walk yet, neither can your bike, you are the only one who can use their legs already so please walk up a few steps alone until I gather my strength and if I can, I'll pick you up again." "OK, I understand, only next time don't put the blame on me," she says and sets off up the steps.

Over-worries

Sometimes we overdo worrying about the whole children thing. Every second baby rattle has a warning that says not for under-threes. Instead of three hours I spend weeks searching for the best child seat on the Internet. I went to school around the corner in a country town, not to Waldorf or Montessori, yet I became a normal person. And despite all that, I spend months stressing about their entrance exams. You can buy a helmet for toddlers that protects their head from bumping into things... I know of at least seven types of water-sandals even though I haven't even looked into the subject. Moreover, I buy them even though I used to love balancing on sharp stones with my bare feet on the shores of Lake Balaton. Is it necessary to immunise against chicken pox? Do we need screening software on the computer? Should the child take a mobile with him when he pops out to the shop around the corner? Is it sufficient to use a factor thirty sunscreen in May or do I need factor fifty?

"In order to have a healthy immune system, a child needs a kilogram of dirt a year" my eighty-year-old pediatrician grandmother enlightens me, as I wash the apple that fell on the floor. Well, at least I don't need to worry about that one. I can buy a dirt pill in the USA.

Play clothes

"Don't sit down there, don't get your trousers dirty" I hear at the playground from some mothers. It makes me think. What am I doing if I take my child to the playground in clothes that shouldn't be soiled? It's a bit like tying his hands together in front of the climbing frame and asking him to climb with his feet and his teeth. I place a barrier in a process designed to let the child gain experience and discover the world freely.

In our family, most clothes are for play because I wouldn't like my children not to be allowed to play anytime anywhere, not only at the playground, but also in the street, in a restaurant, at school. If there are one or two pieces that I'd like to save for special occasions, I only put them on for such events that require nice clothes and then I can ask the children to look after them. However, I shouldn't count on too much care from a two-three-four-five-year-old because children are basically into play, whatever clothes they're wearing.

Guest

A guest in the house, it's often said about children. Guests are polite. Guests are respectful. Guests don't let loose, they behave. I also behave with them even if they're close to my heart. Guests leave and then sometimes I don't hear from them at all for weeks or months. My children are definitely not guests in the house and I wouldn't like for them to be guests either.

Being proactive

I know it, I've experienced it, I've read it, I've learnt it. If there's tension, then the best thing is to be proactive, to attempt to change the rivalling energy into a game of Monopoly, a running contest, wrestling. Add a bit of creativity and whatever it is that they're looking to beat off on each other by winding each other up or hurting one another can come out in a bearable form. I often manage to be proactive and I often don't. In the latter case, I can see how we're speeding, like a fast train, towards an argument. I can't find the brakes and I know that the collision will hurt. I can use this to immerse myself in the I'm-a-crap-mother feeling, while I can also see all the other layers: that it's terribly difficult to be proactive because it takes energy which is often unavailable. It's enough to have had a restless night and that's it. I can't be creative, even if it kills me. Even when I manage to be proactive, it's not always enough to avoid an argument, sometimes it can only be deferred. Like a balloon with more than one hole in it. I put my finger on one hole but the air escapes through another. When steam can only be let off through sibling duels, we still have something to be happy about – let's say, at least there was no blood.

Thumb sucking

I was about eleven when I stopped sucking my thumb. That was twenty-six years ago, but I can still recall the sensation of putting my thumb in my mouth at bedtime and feeling down to my bones that everything was fine, peaceful, and calm, I am safe. What thumb sucking gave me was flow itself.

I was happy that at least one of my five children discovered this self-assuring mechanism. Of course, the stream of comments from left, right, and centre came with it:

"It's very harmful. Why do you let him?"

"He'll need braces, his mouth will become disfigured, his palate will become deformed."

"He won't be able to break the habit."

"His teeth will fall out; his speech will be distorted."

"You should put some chicken bile on his finger."

I've experienced first-hand the difficulties my family had trying to get me to break the habit – and I'm proud of having fought off all attempts. I remember lying next to my cousin after a tiring summer day with the habit-breaking glove-like sack on both of our hands tied strongly to our wrists. We were both convinced that the other one would fail and take off the gloves because she couldn't resist the temptation, but not me, I was strong! I remember how, after a fierce struggle and lots of restless turning, half-asleep, I finally tore that instrument of torture off my hands, forsaking the joy of winning, for that was not half as sweet as the feeling given by my thumb.

Then, eventually, I stopped by myself, of course. When I no longer needed the safety of my thumb, the habit disappeared from my life slowly, unnoticed. My teeth didn't fall out, my mouth didn't become disfigured, and I never needed braces. Even if I had, it's no question which side I would have cheered for at a tooth vs. soul match.

The seven plates

It's 6.30am and there are seven plates in front of me. On one there is some salami, on the next one there is cheese, on the third some bread and butter, on the fourth it's the crust of the bread, on the fifth there's a piece of a Milky Way chocolate bar, on the sixth there are some peppers, on the seventh there's nothing yet. I pause and take a long second to consider how it's possible for her to scream into my face with such a sense of loss and pain on her face when there is so much choice; what can the problem be? Of course, I know that the colour of the last plate is the problem, but I'm a touch irritated by now. I've been jumping up and down without a single word, sweetly handing her the plates and the things to go on them up until now, so at the moment I am a little fed up with, it exhausts me, it creates tension in me.

So, what am I to do?

First – or last, depending on my mental state at the time – for the fraction of a second, I admire childhood existence, the way such deep emotions can be experienced through such a small problem, or at least it is from my point of view. Beautiful. It would require much inner permission for me to be able to scream like her. How wonderful that she has still got all that freedom!

I try to make her see that she is the queen of this huge open buffet and I quickly diagnose that I'm not going to get anywhere on the cognitive level on this occasion. There's little chance of finding a solution along this road to reach the desired state, which is for her to stop screaming so hard that it splits my brain.

When I think this through, I realise instantly that what really bothers me is not that she's screaming, but that she's too close to me, so I tell her that it doesn't matter if she keeps screaming, but it's really bothering me so if she doesn't stop, I shall go into the other room because I can't hear her there.

Then there are times when I start laughing and I hug her. This is rare, but it has happened. Then there are times when I scream with her, funnily, copying her waaaaaaaah. It happens that she's so surprised that she stops.

There is also the case when I reflect on her, not her actions but the feelings and needs I assume she may have: "Are you angry because this is not what you would like?" As soon as I say this I feel it's perfectly understandable, I would like to scream many times when I'm filled with anger. And I tell her this, so she can see that I'm also human – "I understand; it can make me very angry as well when things are not how I'd like them to be."

Even if what's inside her is not exactly what I've guessed, at least we're no longer connecting on the surface on the level of plates, but instead we're examining our feelings. And she will duly say, yes, she's angry or tired.

I make a request: "Please help me by telling me what it is you would like. I understand what it is you wouldn't like, but I don't yet know what you would like, so I don't know how I could help you even though I would like to help."

I'm trying to put myself in her shoes. Why does she need to do this now? Why would I, had I been her? Perhaps this is a game, perhaps she can't find anything better to do and she likes this? If I feel like this, I try to leave the situation on another level: "Come on, let's do a puzzle instead." Sometimes it works. If not, I move on.

Is she testing my boundaries? I try to show her boundaries: go over to the drawer and choose another plate or let's finish having breakfast and go inside.

Then I consider what's inside me. I feel tense from helplessness. I try to say this as well: I'm angry and lost, I can't find a way out of this situation. Displaying myself often brings an opportunity to step out of the situation we're stuck in.

Sometimes, at first I say 'no' to an eighth plate and then she throws a tantrum and amid our battle I change my mind and think, well, why not? But as I'm a believer in consistency, what can I do in such situations? If I relent, it's as if I am giving in to her shouting and her pressure, reinforcing the tantrum by giving her what she wants. She might get the message that if she wants to achieve something, she just needs to scream long enough and hard enough to get it. However, if I refuse to give in, even though inside I've actually changed my mind and relented in my heart, then my child will detect the ambiguity in me, notice me becoming uncertain. To that she will mostly react by fighting harder as my walls are crumbling, and she feels she has a chance, So we have a long and arduous battle ahead. What has worked for me in such instances when I feel ready to give in while she's wailing and demanding, is to say: "Well, I can be convinced but not in that tone" or "Go on, have a good cry and I think afterwards we'll manage to find a solution that suits us both."

In some cases, as I know full well that she would have liked the purple plate, I simply swap the plates. And I also explain at the same time that it would make me feel much better if she asked me nicely to swap them with a 'please', because I function better like that; being spoken to nicely gives me energy the way petrol fuels cars. Or I can say that I've come to a standstill, so I'll go outside and hand her over to her dad.

All these solutions are perfect; the best thing is to do what comes naturally there and then. I frequently have to try three or four different strategies by the time we can navigate ourselves out of the situation – which is solved not by me alone, really, but simply by time.

Swearing day

At the age of eighteen months or two years, it's still considered funny when a child decorates their speech with swearwords. Then, as they grow, it becomes increasingly embarrassing and disturbing.

Why does "fag" sound bad to me when it is okay for others? In my family the word "shit" doesn't shake the ground. Those words that sound bad to me, which consequently, I don't allow my kids to use, will become exciting and much desired by the children; the attraction of taboo is enormous.

So, let them be said! We've established a bad words time, which is only five minutes a month, when everyone can freely say what they want to, let it all come out, give them sound, go on, say it again, more more more, who knows more, who can do fouler, let's compete.

With every single word sounded out, the desire decreases and by the end all taboos lose their attraction. The spoken unspeakables, the sounded-out expletives, take away the tension and don't stay inside to be used in everyday situations.

Yucky

A dead frog? An earwig? Is it ok to touch a slug? Mole poo? In our family, dead animals with meat still on them can only be touched with a stick. All others are free booty. I can't say that I always find it easy to keep to this; I take big breaths when a deer skull is being boiled in the pan or there's a shark-moth hibernating next to the ice cream in the freezer. "Sorry Mama, it's really important for my collection...". Simultaneously they passionately feel sorry for the mother of the moth, as they do have a heart. In our family, yucky is the smell of bananas and things to do with girls.

Should they say sorry?

One child hits the other, the situation is clear-cut, there's a culprit and a victim. I administer justice and tell the guilty party to say sorry. "Say sorry", I tell him. He apologises but for some reason that doesn't appease me. I can't see that he feels remorse, while I feel that there's something not right about the situation. In truth what I'd like him to do is not to just say sorry. I'd like him to understand that it was painful for the other one and I'd like him not to hurt others. I can tell him to apologise or to say that he's sorry, but why? I can't force feelings on him. And what do I achieve by making him say sorry, but he doesn't feel any remorse? If he acts out of compliance, not on his own impulse. If I push him into doing something, I just aggravate the situation. He'll become even more frustrated, which will be taken out on someone, somehow in a few days anyway. I'd like there to be no hurting in the family between children, between adults, and between adults and children. I can and should tell them that. I cannot place expectations on them about how they should or shouldn't feel, but I do have expectations about the way they should and shouldn't behave.

Useful science

As psychology students, we had to read and learn many thousands of pages of descriptions of various experiments. Generally speaking, I concluded that everything is possible and often so is its very opposite. If subjects change as well as other experimental circumstances, the opposite of all basic theses can equally be proven or at least all earlier results that seemed to be set in stone before can be questioned. However, this in no way means that it's useless to run experiments. Quite the opposite, in fact. Pavlov, you dear old master, how much help you give me every single day! I used to run around the flat three or four times in an attempt to round up all the little ants and seat them at the table, needing a considerable amount of quiet and loud words and patience to assist the operation! Then a few years ago I introduced a bell – if there is food, I signal with that. The salivation reflexes set off and the children gather in the kitchen without a single verbal request having to be made.

Words

I like using words. I like showing the world, emotions, thoughts with them. I like the way they can change a situation within a few moments. I like it that I can move the kids' minds, feet, diaphragms with them. I like it that we can come out of a tense situation on some days with a simple instantaneous sorry. I like it that it's possible to love, stroke, and heal with words. I like it that they can be used with the one-week-old as well as the 100-year-old.

One night, it must have been about 8.30 already, the two-and-a-half-year-old was sitting on the toilet crying that she didn't want to pee. "You don't have to, that's fine, if you put a nappy on, just let's move on." I'm merely longing for the end of the day, I don't care who wets themselves and who doesn't. Cleaning teeth, however, is important to me, so I pick her up from the toilet and place her on my lap in order to clean her teeth, where she's screaming with a foaming mouth that she would like to pee. All right, then, I put her back on the loo, but I can sense that I feel like pushing a bit at the end, I feel like throwing her there even – I'm tensing up with anger and helplessness. Words, words, lifesaving, resolving, helping, shifting words, well I can't find these anywhere now. So, I hug my obnoxiously wailing child and both her and me relax into the long and tight embrace, then we both move towards the bed, dull and silent. I like it that words are of no use to me at all sometimes.

Hugging

What I like about hugging is that it's such a simple thing, yet it can create truly deep moments of connection in a variety of situations. When I feel that my child is invisibly far from me, a hug can bring us close within a fraction of a second. If I can go and hug him during or after a painful argument, we can both save ourselves hours of pain. When I cannot comfort him with my words, thirty seconds of tight hugging can dry up his tears. I hug him when something hurts, I hug him when he's happy, I hug him when we're making up, I hug him anyway. The sensation of his scent and heartbeat highlights the essence of it all in a nanosecond: we're there for each other.

Balls matter

Anything that is round is attractive. To throw, to kick, to hit the other with, to aim at the bin. The flat is small, windows have been broken. It's also loud – I have plenty of reasons to feel irritated by the kids playing with balls inside. Equally, it would be great if they could play with balls inside. So, I buy ones that can be tied on and kicked about. Table tennis in the store room, basketball hoop in the garden. I sign some of them up for football training. It's still not enough. There's still not a single day I don't have to tell someone off.

So, unfortunately, I'll have to work on the fact that it bothers me then. It's not my aim not to mind at all, just not to let it irritate me quite so much. I'm on trial at the moment: they can play with a ball and I'm working on myself.

Spoilt kids

Sometimes I say to them: "You children are spoilt, you don't know how good you have it!" Even if there is some truth in this, it doesn't seem like a good thing to say. I don't feel it's fair, but why?

They don't know, because I haven't taken them to visit a

family living below the poverty line, and they haven't been starved for even half a day. They don't know because they work the way a normal healthy person does: the brain ceases to respond to identical and regular stimuli. We become habituated, to use the psychological term. We get used to the good stimuli. We get used to the sound of the train, to smells – the train driver does not hear the noise of the train, the dentist does not smell the surgery. It's harder to see the beauty of the city where I walk every day. Yet I can feel amazed by the sweet smell of my child after spending a few hours apart.

I know this with my brain, but it doesn't change the fact that it bothers me when my children don't appreciate the everyday goodness. So, I look for techniques. I tell them that sometimes I walk around the city imagining that I'm a tourist. Wow, it must be brilliant to live here, where the city is sliced into two by a river. I look higher up at the houses from the tram instead of keeping my eyes on street level as usual – and wow, what a beautiful façade this building has! We've played the same game together at home: look at all those books, all those toys, and gee, a bearded dragon. Just how lucky the child who can keep a bearded dragon must be! It's pretty cool that you can draw on the wall in this flat... Waiting for the bus at the bus stop, instead of counting the minutes till the bus comes, we count how many different sounds we can hear at the same time: birds, people, the street, the rain, somebody shouting, the wind blowing – what an exciting world!

The other day one of my sons said that he didn't think it was true that every cloud had a silver lining. So, we played a game: he said something bad or something good and I pointed out the not necessarily obvious aspects then we swapped roles. He started off with a difficult one: "What's good about great-grandfather dying?" "We inherited a huge television," I replied immediately. He was astonished by my response. I carried on explaining that many people think that there are things such as death, for example, that are one-dimensionally sad. Even if it does bring something good, it's not polite to mention it. I believe it's much better not to create taboos, but talk things through openly. I've seen children and adults often relieved just by speaking about the unspeakable. At the same time, the initial aspect remains true – I don't feel any less sad about someone's death just because I notice something good his passing has brought about. This search for different aspects enthused the children. It was exciting and funny and helped us see everyday stuff in more complex layers. Such games can also show the beauty and value of our present life without the need for an illness or a tragedy – and you don't even have to be a grown-up to see them.

Making friends

When my child finds a friend at nursery, a real close friend whom he would like to meet outside playgroup as well, a friend he wants to spend time with at the weekend too, well, that's something to be happy about. When I observe his interactions mostly with family members, I tend to see him too closely emotionally, and some details can only be seen from further away. I can delight in seeing his world opening up, in seeing that there's someone important to him apart from members of the family, the way he can laugh, feel at ease with and build a relationship with someone. Years of parental input can be detected in crumbs, traces, moves, half sentences. And when he's arguing, I can be glad that he's not doing it with me.

PS: If the parents of the chosen friend are bearable, that's good fortune. If they are actually amiable, well, that's a gift from God.

Consumables

I've put seas of patience, sky-high amounts of time, thousands of years' worth of energy and attention into some of the issues that don't shift from that spot where they feel so uncomfortable. One of these, for example, is underwear and socks finding their way to the laundry. I've asked nicely countless times. I've begged, I've reasoned, I've made it transparent why this so bothers me. I've argued about it calmly and in a raised voice and I've tried shouting. We have been around the issue a thousand times from a thousand different angles, like a dog around a bitch in heat. There's a result. Some of the kids don't have to be told, some don't always have to be reminded, but there's not a single day that I don't find at least one sock, more like three or four on average, hiding under the carpet. I'm running out of options and all this helplessness breeds anger in me.

But I won't give up. When I try to remove a screw and I've had a go with the small screwdriver, the star screwdriver, the red one, the electric one, but none of them do the job, that doesn't mean that the screw is unscrewable or the screwdrivers don't work. If it's important for me that it's unscrewed, I'll look it up on the Internet or call a friend or an expert to help. Or I might decide to hit the screw with a hammer from the other side, even if I don't want to go for this option for fear of damaging the material it's in. So, at the moment, it's a hundred forints for each piece of clothing left lying around. They either

135

get used to throwing everything in the laundry, or I'll get rich, or we'll find another way.

Sex education

I don't remember my parents ever giving me sex education talks; the subject was somehow rather naturally a part of our everyday lives.

As much as I like showering on my own, it does happen that I consider it safer to have my two-year-old there with me. It's natural that he asks questions about what he can see on my body, about things he has on his body as well and ones he doesn't and ones I don't and about what all of those bits can be used for. Sometimes the four-year-old comes in as well, because even though she's fine playing outside, she urgently needs to know whether Superman has a brother and I don't grab for the towel to cover myself. Of course, the seven-year-old no longer sits on the side of the bath and the time comes when situations in which they see me naked become rare. And the time also comes when they send me out of the bathroom. But I still don't go to a separate room to breastfeed my youngest in order to hide my breasts from the older ones.

Children usually ask only as much as they are ready to take in. I don't start listing the different lovemaking positions when the four-year-old asks me how children are made, but I do tell them without any aversions or masking about the fact that it requires a man putting his willy into a woman's vagina. I try to sense with my feelers how much information is easily digestible. I observe their tone of voice, I await their questions, and I stop the exchange of information if they signal somehow that it was enough – for example, by rolling around the floor in laughter.

It's the evening, it's past story time, the lights are off, it's dark and one of the teenagers asks me whether people in films really kiss. Then from this question on there's no stopping them. One enquiry leads to the next, there are no boundaries, a hard half-hour follows. I'm not saying that while feeding my youngest I easily find the words for what is good in breastfeeding or how gay men make love, but at the same time I'm glad to receive all questions. And finally, I also feel happy when after the discussion they announce that they are ready to sleep now, because even talking about sex is ever so exhausting.

In a minute

I'll change you in a minute, I'll feed you in a minute, we'll get there in a minute, I'll put the phone down in a minute, dinner will be ready in a minute – in a minute, in a minute, in a minute, I tell him a hundred times a day from his birth. I'll clean my teeth in a minute, I'll go and have my bath in a minute, I'm coming to have dinner in a minute, he tells me from about the age of two. He's learnt superbly from me. Sometimes a minute does mean a minute for me or for them, but sometimes it can mean ten, and they use it exactly the way I do – with the difference being that it is fine when I use it and annoying when they do...

With my fourth child, I start an experiment. She's only a few months old when I begin to navigate my in-a-minutes with more accuracy: when it really is just a minute, I use it, but when it's probably more, I say two minutes and if it's even more, I say five, six, or ten. I change some of my in-a-minutes to specific points of reference, such as after I've cut the meat, after I've been to the toilet, after I've made a phone call – and I make sure I adhere to these. This way, it's much clearer for them when they'll get what they would like. And when she says she'll listen to that piece of music and then she'll come, she really does, she keeps her word. I find that this clearer communication is more predictable for me, so it's safer and more reliable and the children probably feel exactly the same.

Wish fulfillment

When he's born, when he's a few days old, when he's a few weeks old, a few months old, it's obvious to me that as far as possible I try to fulfill all his desires. A newborn cannot be spoilt, as the part of his brain responsible for manipulation has not yet developed. By picking him up, breastfeeding him thirty times a day, he'll not be spoilt, he'll just feel safe in the world. If the consequence of his crying is that the people around him do something for him, it'll be his experience, his innate knowledge that it's worth wishing and trying to express his desires because it influences what happens to him.

Oh, yes, but then he grows, the sweet little darling, and luckily so does his brain. The period of testing boundaries arrives, and can last for as long as fifteen years, when it's also my job to show him how far and no further. Meanwhile, I'd like him to hold on to his ability to desire, not to cripple his ambition to devour the world. But if I give him everything all the time, my ten-year-old will be spoilt according to my definition, which irritates me and this benefits neither of us.

So where do I draw the line? How far can he go, how far should I go, what should I allow and what should I not? I can't do anything but listen inwardly and pinpoint my fears; refine my hearing and my soul-sniffers; scan where the given child's current wish stems from and what me fulfilling it would result in and what happens if I do nothing. I weigh up every single case separately. I decide, listening inwardly, whether I should try to satisfy. I do a lot in many cases and I also decide many times not to do anything at the time. It's a pleasure to occasionally come across desires which are impossible for me to fulfill and I can say no straight away. The wonder of simplicity. I believe that there need to be unfulfilled yearnings because they take you forward, they can transform into different dreams and can stay with you even to adulthood.

For years, I longed for a barking plastic dog, and I didn't get it – then ten years later I got a real one. Sometimes it happens that I'd like to give them what they desire, but not right away. Because I'd like to wait for the wish to grow, to let him feel it more intensely, to let him mention five times a day how much he'd like to read a particular book, even when I've bought it already. I like to sense the best time for giving, for fulfilling a wish. If I'm lucky, I manage to do it before he borrows the book from his friend. Sometimes I overdo it. I keep collecting stickers for him in secret so that I can give him fifteen packs all at once for effect and he's given thirty packs by his school friend. I view such instances as a failure, they feel bad, for in this case my fifteen packs do not hit the intended spot. But that should be the least of our problems. He will have plenty of desires yet and I'll get plenty of opportunities to play with wish (un)fulfillment.

Keeping secrets

Keeping secrets is an important and good thing. We train children from an early age to enable them to do so. The eighteen-month-old already plays with doing things he's not allowed to in secret: he sees the marble on the floor, looks at me, and grabs the marble with the speed of lightning, turns away, puts it in his mouth, takes it out, hides it behind his back, looks at me again and laughs. My reaction is interesting to him. He laughs at me and does it again.

The two-year-old and I shop together for a present for her brother. We have a discussion about not telling him about the surprise. She draws for birthdays and we keep a secret about what she drew and where we hid the drawing. She giggles with her hand over her mouth and asks a thousand times – this is such an exciting place for her, as if we're playing hide and seek in Mirrorland.

At the age of three, he hides my mobile phone under his pillow as a joke and doesn't tell me where it is when I'm searching for it. He creates secrets and tests how far they're exciting and interesting and at which point I get angry about them. At the age of four to five, he convinces his brother or sister not to tell me that they have found the secret chocolate stash in the drawer and have eaten it.

We experience the essence of secrets slowly, savouring it. Their true nature takes years to evolve in us. There are good and bad secrets and there are grey areas. If we keep quiet about a surprise, that's OK, but can we go as far as telling a lie? When I've already bought my child a book, but haven't given it to him yet and he suddenly comes up with the idea of spending his savings on that very book, what do I do? Do I say, for example, that it can no longer be bought at the shop, they've run out? I don't like telling a lie, not even with good intent; I'd rather choose the half-truth as a solution. I tell him to hold on to his money a little longer and think over whether this is really what he'd like to spend it on. A child can't know exactly what good intent is; even in adulthood it's often a philosophical question. I'd like them to be able to trust my word and for this reason, whenever it's possible, I must tell the truth. For later, when they have a secret, I'd like them not to lie. I'd like them to be able to say that they don't want to tell me, or, with what they consider good intent, to divert with a half-truth. Because if they lie, my faith in them wobbles too.

And then there are those bad secrets. When he's convinced by his mate to do something that's unpleasant for him and not to tell anyone about it. Or when he steals money from my purse. Or even worse, when a family member or someone he knows, or a teacher, strokes his bottom and tells him not to talk to mummy about that because she would be angry. From the two-year-old to the teenager, I keep repeating that those secrets that make them feel bad in their skin, those that make them stressed, those that make them feel uncomfortably tense or sad, well those are the secrets that don't have to be kept but need to be revealed hastily to someone they trust.

Leave them be

I give time for the family to get familiar with the new family member. Some will be jealous, some will want to gain attention with the odd tantrum, some will have a cough for weeks, some don't even need a single day to accept the new situation.

I let them have the time to learn to sit. Some sit up at the age of six months, others are a year old when they learn. I give myself time to find my way back into my body. It took nine months to change shape one way, so it's not going to be a matter of two weeks to get back to the way I feel comfortable. I let them cry, be angry, have a laughing fit – I allow all tension, hurt, sadness, and joy to come out. I let them go up the stairs in their own rhythm. I let them run or stop if they're tired. I even let them take a step back. I let them cling to me, distance themselves, go off, come back. I leave them alone, let them be. I let them make mistakes, I let them correct them. I leave them be and I let me be, too.

6

Self-knowledge
as a tool

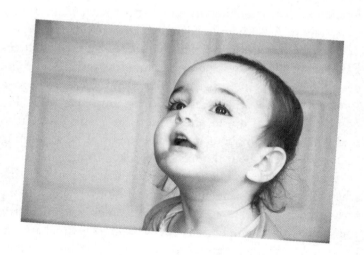

Be they small or big, children or adults, if there's a conflict between us, isn't it simpler to see the other party as the source of it?! Perhaps the circumstances, the situation, fate, God, their parents or mine, my ex or his new wife, the state, and society can also be added to the picture. The reason it is so much better to only see these (also valid and existing) layers of the conflict is because then I don't need to dig into my own depths, I avoid tearing open my wounds. Ever so much simpler, a more pain-free life.

No matter how unpleasant the process can be, mostly it works better for me in the long term when I can make a shift inside, when I'm able to find my own sticking point, and start looking at that, scratching it, applying the glue, taking things apart, and making them fit back together in a different way.

No, this does not mean that I'm the reason my daughter's PE kit didn't find its way home and into the washing machine over the past six months. If I'm looking for a scapegoat, someone to blame, that doesn't take me anywhere at all. The point of change is not to pronounce whose fault it is, but to find what I can do about it and that tends to be something that's very rarely about the specific problem itself.

Seriously, why would it bother me that her socks stink when I'm not the one smelling them?! If I look deeper into my feelings, using self-knowledge, I can come up with nice little soundbites, for example: what my relationship to shame is, the question of perfection, living up to expectations, making judgements, being in control. Self-knowledge as a tool is an invisible, universal toolkit. There's no bolt that cannot be adjusted with it, no crack that cannot be filled, no rust that it cannot get rid of, no cogwheel it can't start turning again.

Mornings

"Wake-up time, good morning, get up, time to get out of bed, get ready, go on, please, clean your teeth, have you packed everything? It's Thursday, have you got your swimming kit as well? Don't forget your sandwiches! We're late. You're late. I'm late!" I drive them like horses, lashing at them with the whip of my words.

I'm looking, searching in myself for the reason I get repeatedly stressed in the mornings. I don't believe that the children are innocent; I think they also play a part in our recurrent working patterns, but I prefer to find the place for change in myself.

First of all, I swear that as of the next day, I'll be a good mother, patient, non-shouting, non-driving. Sometimes I manage it. Then the following day I fail. Many times I succeed, but it's unpredictable when it'll work and when it won't, so this doesn't make for a perfect solution.

I'm looking for the hidden layers in this seemingly simple, recurrent, and disturbing episode. I can see my own learned patterns in my mornings: when I was small, according to my mother, the beginning of the day was often difficult, and we were frequently in a hurry.

I notice that when I'm in the room and say, "wake up" every minute, they stay in bed for much longer than when I say it only once and then leave. I let them sense whether we're actually on time.

I stop saying that they'll be late. I just ask whether they'd like to be on time. I hated being late. It made me feel uncomfortable when the teacher told me off. I missed it when I didn't have a few minutes to have a laugh with the others before the school bell rang. Do you like that? No? Then do something about it. I can't leave on time for you. When they're at school, they're old enough to understand and take responsibility for their own part.

I stop saying that they should hurry up; I say it only when it's really necessary, and even then, I just say it once or twice.

I stop saying that I'll leave without them. I only do so if I really will leave without them, if they're big enough to go to school alone. In any other case they know that I'm just trying to scare them and thus I disintegrate my own integrity.

I can also see that I wake them up at the very last moment to let the poor tired children sleep as much as possible. I intend to look out for them by doing so, but perhaps I'm being overprotective. As soon as I realise this, my next question follows: do I achieve more by letting them sleep fifteen minutes longer, or by having a stress-free morning? There's no question. By identifying and shifting my own inner layers, we've managed to establish quality mornings from one day to the next.

Grade C

My older sons like to get good grades. I can understand that, I used to be the same. However, this also means that they really don't like getting bad grades. Which is partly brilliant, because they're motivated, though I'd like them not to take it so much to heart when something doesn't turn out as expected.

So, where am I in all of this? I keep telling them that it's perfectly fine to get the occasional grade C, but I don't feel that I can fully cope with the actual situation.

What can I do for this to change? Partly I keep reassuring

them on the level of words that it's ok with me when they get the occasional grade C, and partly I make it transparent to them that sometimes I discover a little knot in my stomach, too, when faced with lower grades, but I'd like to change this. It's not about them, I think, but it's probably down to my compulsion to please.

So how can I move acceptance down to gut level, so it can really be me and not just a sentence I say? For example, by noticing different aspects through the children. When they come home and say that they got a grade C, but it would've been an A, had they put down what they'd thought instead of listening to their classmate who whispered the wrong answer to them, finally there is an example for us both about what a lower grade can teach us: it's worth trusting yourself and listening inwardly. Finally, something tangible. Finally, something that can be experienced, something that shifts things in me too. It's never too late to unwrap my responsible child-self and mould her.

Transparency

He can say he's hungry or tired even in the middle of a fit. This is wonderful because it means that even a two-year-old is able to move out of our games, our reoccurring patterns, and that I'm not the only one responsible.

For a long time, I thought that I put a burden on my children by telling them what was going on inside me, that I was tired or irritable and impatient because I'd had a hard day, because let's say I'd had to queue at the post office and I'd got upset about it. Then I realised that I was only fooling myself when I imagined that I'd be putting a burden on them by explaining what was going on inside me, as they could accurately tell that for some reason I was off-centre. By not telling them the cause of my discomfort, they took it on themselves and believed that they might be the reason, whereas by telling them, I make it transparent and it all falls into place for them as well. And the same for me, when they can tell me about what's going on for them.

As an adult, I also experience similar situations. For example, I meet a friend I haven't seen in a while and I can see that she's distracted, I can feel that she's not really there, she's asking me superficial questions, she's not listening to my answers, she's fidgeting with her phone. What am I thinking? She doesn't feel like talking to me? She doesn't want to be friends anymore? She's angry with me for some reason? And then she suddenly tells me that she's had an argument with her mother that morning and she feels really upset about that. What will the result be? I instantly feel relieved and can connect with her. I feel empathy, I start asking her about details – and a real, attentive exchange may ensue. My child experiences exactly the same when I'm invisible and when I make myself transparent to him.

Of course, the extremes are strange here as well. For example, when I'm telling the six-month-old that I'm feeling tense because I've had a disagreement with the neighbour. But it's still worth it: I feel better by explaining which, in turn, can only benefit my child.

It's not only solving the actual situation that makes this approach worthwhile; it's also because by doing so, I provide a pattern. It's elevating to see my child using this communication technique with others. One day my ten-year-old had a huge fight with his brother and he was really cruel to him. After circling the flat, he sat down next to his brother and said to him: "I've noticed that when I've had a bad day at school, I can best take it out on you, even if you haven't done anything wrong at all."

Expectations

Even before the birth, I have expectations of my child: it would be good if it were a boy, or a girl; I'd like them to have blue eyes like me, to be born easily and on time, and especially, to be healthy. When he's born, he should be able to feed straight away, sleep through the night, not have colic or cry a lot… in short, I'd like him be user-friendly. Then all he has to do is develop nicely inside and out.

My child is unable to fulfill all this, no matter how cool, clever, beautiful and perfect he is. The point in question is whether I put things as desires or expectations. Desires are about me alone while expectations are also up to him. I want an easy birth – OK, that's a desire. He shouldn't have colic, he shouldn't cry – these are expectations. However, if I rephrase it more carefully I can transform it into a wish: I hope I won't have to walk up and down with my baby at night. More precisely: I want my life to be free of difficulty.

I can't expect anything of my child that he cannot influence, either when he's a baby or later on. When he's tiny, it's easy to distinguish between situations he can affect and ones he can't. In the beginning, he can do nothing about anything but week by week this changes until by the time he's an adult he's fully responsible for his actions. I expect the two-year-old, for instance, to go to sleep even though I shouldn't, as falling asleep isn't a matter of making a decision. I can only really expect him to do things that take him towards going to sleep: lie down, close his eyes, don't talk, please. I can't expect a schoolchild to get better grades, as it's the teacher who gives the grades, so it's not the child alone who's responsible for them. What I can expect is that he studies more, pays attention in the lessons, and does all his homework.

I can expect things at his level of actions, as managing those is in his hands. And if I can transform my expectations into desires, then I often take huge loads off my child's shoulders – as well as finding out things about myself, too.

Giving

What's the difference between giving with joy, giving for approval, giving out of fear or expectation, or giving to avoid feeling ashamed? My actions are motivated by my desires, my quest for joy, to experience happiness, but my behaviour is also influenced by negative feelings such as fear or the wish to avoid shame. If I give something with a good feeling, be that food, hugs, or attention, the one I'm giving to can sense the purity of that. If I give because I want to live up to expectations, to do favours, or out of fear or shame, the whole affair becomes tainted; there'll be something invisible but detectable about it. And from that point on, things slip.

If I hate having to cook every day, if I never do it out of joy, then the inner tension caused by wanting to live up to expectations creates anger and sentences such as these will follow: "You never thank me for making a sacrifice for you every single day!" "I slog my guts out every day like a servant while you keep staring at the TV screen with your feet up." The role of a martyr poisons inconspicuously. It's never too late to pinpoint the things I do without pleasure; there's no deadline or age limit for identifying them and making a change. And that doesn't mean I should do things fundamentally differently. I don't have to go for the other extreme, for example, by not making food at all or only eating takeaways. I can make food, but it can often be pizza or salad, so I move towards the easier options and can perhaps move away from not giving wholeheartedly. Consequently, I remove myself from the role of a martyr as well. Thus, I can actually give more than I would give with a two-course dinner.

No question questions

As a mother, I often ask no-question questions. This is when the enquirer is not really interested in the answer, the question does not stem from curiosity, but is used to express some form of criticism. For example, when I ask my children "Haven't you cleaned your teeth yet?" I am not looking for the response "No". I actually mean "I'd really like you to clean your teeth as soon as possible." When my mother-in-law asks me, with my seven-month-old in her arms, "Does he eat any proper food or is he still only on breastmilk?" it's not a question either, as she's fully aware that the answer is no. It's a criticism wrapped in a question. When I ask my husband "Are you going to be back as late again tonight as you were last night?" this may be a covert reproach about him failing to get home the night before as early as I'd have liked him to.

I try my best to really ask a question when I ask a question and, in an attempt to create a deeper connection, I try to react to the non-questions put to me not as real questions. So, I tend to say to my children "Go and clean your teeth, please."

151

I try to communicate to my husband clearly that I feel really tired by 6pm and I usually hit rock bottom around about that time, so it would mean a lot to me if he could manage his day so he can get home by then. And as for my mother-in-law, I try to enquire: "Yes, he's on breastmilk, but do you actually mean to say that you feel concerned that he's not eating solids yet?" And as for myself, I try to ask real questions, not ones like "Why can't I be a more patient mother to the kids?" For this is not a question either, but me having a go at myself.

Guilty

I shouted at my child – crack the whip! I left him to cry for two minutes – what kind of a mother does that? I'd no strength left, yet again – hell and damnation!

To accept myself as fallible, as someone who makes mistakes, as someone who's not perfect, is a far tougher job than bathing in guilt. With guilt, however, I achieve nothing apart from walking around in circles, making me feel dizzier and more and more scared and depressed. I relive bad feelings over and over again, but it doesn't take me forward. Just like keeping the shoes that I used to love but have grown out of: even though they continuously hurt my feet, I still can't get rid of them.

One of the worst feelings for me is when I lose my patience and anger pours out of me in the form of shouting. It's scary to see the fear in my children's eyes, the same fear I experienced as a child when I was being shouted at. At the point at which I feel how I'm about to behave, I'm already flooded by feelings of guilt even though I haven't even said the words or raised my voice. However, I also feel unable to stop myself, like a river overflowing its bed. On the one hand, I'm trying to step out of my guilt trip and look for the solution in myself, to notice what I could do differently, while on the other I'm trying to accept that sometimes I just can't do better and that in itself doesn't constitute a major catastrophe. My child is not going to see a psychologist because I shout at him, unless this is my dominant form of relating to him. He's not going to turn to mind-altering drugs instead of friends to help him in times of difficulty just because I smoked two cigarettes over the course of nine months of pregnancy. He's not going to be unhappy or get a divorce because I leave the unhappy relationship I'm in with his father.

Guilt is good. It highlights my blocks perfectly: limitations which, if shifted, can enable me to have a happier life. I always act the best way I can, give the most of what I can give at the time. By accepting my faults and my failings, the whole picture in the end will look all right to me. This way I can be more certain that I'm doing okay than by being immersed in guilt. In the latter case, not only do I burden myself, and consequently my children, with my failings, but also with my own guilt.

The why game

My two-year-old has entered the why phase. Anyone who has ever lived through this knows full well that the endless questions can lead to moments of frustration. The reasons why we should answer all our children's questions patiently can be read about in thousands of places: to help their intellectual abilities develop, to keep them open to the world, to give them attention, and so on. And I can learn a lot from it and from them. I can use this tool to discover myself, to identify my own feelings, motivation, desires, fixations, sore points. I don't need to do anything other than the very thing my child does: start off with a seemingly weightless problem and keep asking why again and again. It's important that just the same way my child ignores that I'm getting fed up with their questions, I should also refuse to leave myself alone and keep going until I discover a point of sensitivity (giving me satisfaction, an aha moment, or pain), which I will feel in my stomach. I'll be tingling with joy or feel stabbed by sadness or be flooded by feelings of shame or anger – I'll usually be able to get to an intense feeling if I manage to give myself honest and deep answers.

I don't feel like cooking today. Why? Because I have no idea what to cook. Why? Because I find it tiring that I have to come up with something new every day. Why? Because I'm tired of it, I'd rather go to the cinema. Why? Because I enjoy going to the cinema but unfortunately, I don't have the time these days. Why? Because I spend my time doing other things. Why? Because I give urgent tasks higher priority and leave my own recharging options till last. Why? Perhaps because I'd feel guilty if there was no lunch and I'd gone to the cinema instead. Why? Because I'd feel that I'm not a good mum. Why? Because it seems to be set in me like concrete that a good mother puts caring for her loved ones above anything else and I can't shift from this. Why?

Entrance exams

I never thought that worrying about an entrance exam could be so stressful. Meanwhile I keep saying to myself and to the children, too, that no matter what the result is, it'll be just fine and that we'll figure out how they can find their happiness. I believe as well as know that it's the search that's really important, but on an emotional level, this certain belief is accompanied by an IKEA shopping bag full of anxiety. I hate feeling my stomach in a knot, I hate that it squashes me and paralyzes my soul.

The moment comes when I realise that I'm more anxious than they are. And then I realise that this is pointless and the one thing I'm definitely not doing is helping them. We'll sink together if they don't keep me afloat, which is not too healthy in the long term either.

So, I remove myself from this symbiotic state and start looking for my own centre, my own security, my inner balance. I shift to positive experiences. I watch the blossoming trees, listen to music, meet friends, exercise for twenty minutes. Not much later, I'm able to think, when hearing the sounds of my smaller children's uninhibited play, how sweet they are instead of thinking "Lucky them, so carefree at this age but when they get to the stage their older brothers are at right now...". When I look at my children going through the weeks before the entrance exams, my stomach no longer ties in a knot. Now I notice how much they enjoy their food, how happily they go training, and how intensely they throw themselves into reading a good book, even on their most difficult days. And then instead of worrying, I'm flooded with pride: the way they choose solidarity instead of cracking under pressure, coloured with lots of laughter and their frequent squabbles, much preferred to anxiety. I notice in them and simultaneously in myself and in our life together those details that energise us, all of which must have been there all the time and I was just unable to see them in my limited state of consciousness. And with these small steps, finding the way back to myself fairly quickly, I become a mother capable of giving support yet again.

Changes

Starting nursery, going to secondary school, weaning... phew, the big changes of different ages. What they all have in common is my question to myself about whether I'm ready. Am I ready to let them go? Am I ready to go back to work? Am I completely ready for this new phase? Am I ready to let go of all that I enjoyed in the previous one? Am I ready to see the new phase as an adventure? Am I ready to make new connections or renew the old ones? Am I ready to cope in a new environment? Am I ready to take a new road instead of the usual one to the playground? Am I ready to let go of those good times of being together?

I ask myself these questions and nibble through them, round and round like an apple looking for the seeds inside. Just like them at the age of three or thirteen, I, too, can feel at the age of thirty-seven that I'm losing something, that I'm afraid of new things, of the unknown.

My last three years were filled with being with children. It was sometimes like this, sometimes like that. It was easy as well as hard, but I'm certain that I liked it. Even if I know that in starting nursery I won't lose my child, I'll definitely lose part of her. I have to grieve for and let go of the period when we spent day and night together. I've already found the issue I have to work with here. I'm able to move towards solutions and not think in extremes. I can look for the possibilities, for example, when I can temporarily create a schedule whereby she doesn't spend eight hours a day at nursery but has a few mornings off, just like she's done until now. If I can pick her up after lunch a couple of times, or I can arrange a mummy's day every two months, I don't see the situation as being so dire.

I tell the adolescent that secondary school will surely be brilliant even though they won't get home for lunch and we'll see much less of each other. OK, I have an issue with the fact that we'll see less of each other. I tell him that I'm afraid we'll lose some of our connection, laughing together. I'm worried I'll hardly ever see him. He hugs me. That's much better. The arrival of a new period has already become more acceptable, I'm less afraid. And, incidentally, he also tells me that he's worried, too. So, an important, deep moment of very real heart-to-heart connection is born.

"I've been breastfeeding you for nearly three years, you're a big girl now," I tell my daughter.

"I'm not big."

"Ok, then maybe I feel that it's too much for me."

"Fine," she says.

I haven't made much progress. Perhaps I haven't managed to make my feelings clear. When I succeed, I often feel a sense of relief, but not this time. OK, I carry on.

"It's getting too much for me to feed both you and your brother, it's often uncomfortable, it sometimes hurts. I can see that it is terribly important to you and I wouldn't like to do anything bad for you, but I wouldn't like to do anything that's bad for me either."

"Then will you tell me a story instead sometimes and I'll cuddle up, is that OK?"

Yes, now I can feel that something has started, even if it's just in her head, I don't need more than this right now.

The changes expected but not yet completed in our lives

can bring feelings of uncertainty. Then, when the new makes its presence felt, we're no longer left grieving for the old, but can hold onto the great and not-so-great new things.

Literally

"You're going to kindergarten after the summer!" She's crying, blubbering. She must be anxious. Separation is hard for her. Oh, my poor little thing must be fretting that I won't be by her side. She must be thinking that she'll be missing her brother or she's worrying about what the teacher is going to be like.

"What's the matter?" I ask, giving her the opportunity to choose the most appealing one from the above list of causes for anxiety. After all there is freedom of emotions in our family.

"How am I going to get there? How will I be able to go to nursery when I'm still little and I can't walk the streets alone?" I have a good laugh – at myself. All right, I get it. I'll pay more attention to the literal meaning of my words for one, and for another, instead of projecting, I'll examine my own feelings more closely....

The power of words

I was two and a half, talking, and nappy-free at night when my grandfather died. I asked my mother why he was no longer alive. She replied, "He couldn't pee", translating kidney dysfunction into child language.

The answer we'd been unable to find for twenty years became clear a few years ago from the diary my mother had kept about us: it was after this response that I started wetting myself at nights and carried on doing so to the age of 11. Because who the hell wants to die just because they can't pee?

Shall I solve his problems?

Have you heard the joke about when Maurice turns to his mother at half past seven in the morning telling her that he has to take an object from the 1980s to school and he also needs a four-line poem about a blackbird? No, this is not a joke.

Do I solve his problem? At first blink I look at how I'm feeling at the time. If I say, "this keeps happening" or "you always do this" or "you never blah blah", if I communicate about him, we'll probably end up having an argument. If I'm able to say that I feel under pressure when we're leaving for school, so I'm talking about myself, then the whole thing won't feel so bitter. I can still decide whether to do the homework or not. It helps if I tell him the reason for my decision, so he can understand it/me as well. Perhaps it's against my principles to take over his tasks, but it's also possible that I've done way too much homework in my life already and I don't feel like doing any more. There are times when I'll gladly do it for him because I feel like it.

Is it unquestionably helpful if I sort things out for him? At the given moment, it definitely is, but what about in the long term? Am I afraid that if I help him now, he'll get lazy and leave everything to the last minute and to me? Am I concerned that by supporting him too much, he'll not learn to solve his own problems? If I feel any question arising in me, I'll find some feelings behind them and if I share those, it opens up more ways, so there are more options on offer to help us move towards solutions rather than tensions. My feelings cannot be argued with, and he can also show his own feelings far more easily – colour on colour, suit on suit.

Re-labelling

"Have you done your homework yet?" I ask at 8pm. "I haven't had time" replies the schoolboy, who has been at home for four hours.

Children are not born with this sentence ready to use. They must have learnt it from someone, and that someone is most likely to be me. I haven't had time to sew a button on my trousers for the past eleven months. I haven't had time to sell the cookbooks collecting dust in the house for the past year and a half. I haven't had time to call the dentist for three months and I haven't had time to read a book for weeks. I can preach to my children that they have time for what they make time for, or I can act in a way that they can copy instead of the "I haven't had time" rhetoric. I begin to shine a light on my everyday actions and identify the things I say I don't have time for. And I re-label them. Some I re-label as things I don't want to devote time to, some make it to my "things to do" file. More specifically, I have written to two people I've been putting off writing to. I've asked for an appointment at the dentist's. I've moved the stuff that needs sewing from the study to somewhere more noticeable. I realised that I didn't have time to sell the cookbooks on the Internet, so I took them to a charity – and I did the same with the clothes the kids have grown out of. This inner tidy-up has resulted in a new orderliness, unseen for a long time, in the study as well.

But it gave me an even better feeling to tell my son what greater good he has actually managed to do by telling me he hadn't had time to do his homework.

My longings

I'm longing to reach the age when nobody has to be put to sleep and simultaneously for them to stay small so that I can feel their breath on me when putting them to sleep. I'm longing to never breastfeed again while at the same time I'm also wishing for this period of cuddling up for a breastfeed to last. I'm longing to hear the one-year-old speak and also for him to communicate only without words. I'm longing for my big children to hang out with their friends, yet I wish that they'd come home straight after school. I'm longing for them to go to college and then university, to separate, while I also wish that they'd stay close.

I may have conflicting desires, but often they only seem to be conflicting. When I unfold them, and look at the layers one by one, if I phrase it to myself more precisely, it's easier to see what it is that I'd really like.

I like the closeness in breastfeeding, but not that I have to get my breast out, or even say no, when it's required by my baby. I can hold on to the closeness by telling a story with my child sitting on my lap and I can also look for the opportunity to cuddle up in various situations.

I long for them to hang out with their friends because I'd like them to experience all the joys and excitement of social living. But I wouldn't like to lose my connection with them, so I'd be happy if they could talk to me, share with me some of the things going on inside them.

By elaborating on my longings, I see that one doesn't exclude the other. I'm more likely to be able to fulfill my desire, possibly even more than one, if I can also communicate outwardly with more precision. It doesn't have to be wrapped up in child language; it can be said just the way I put it to myself.

Communicating feelings/desires

If I say "Put down the toilet seat. I can't believe you can't even do something as simple as that," then I really just call the other person into battle, I start a fight. If I say, "When I see the toilet seat up, I feel tense because I don't like having to put it down myself," then I'm talking about myself. My feelings and my desires cannot be faulted. Saying "I'd like to spend more time with just the two of us," rarely warrants a response like "What stupid things you long for, is that really your biggest problem?"

However, it's not the words used to express desire that make something into a desire. Saying "I wish you'd put the toilet seat down" is not a desire, it's an expectation. Just like saying "I feel that you're aggressive" is not a feeling, it's labelling. Things like these take me forward: "I wish we wouldn't fight so much about the toilet seat thing," or "When you raise your voice, I feel frightened."

Of course, written down like this it all seems so simple and straightforward, but in the situation, when the feelings in my stomach swell to rise above my level of consciousness and I begin to use my usual and much-tried mechanisms with greater intensity, the whole thing is made much harder. It takes mostly inner security (more simply, feeling good in my own skin) not to label the other party but to talk about myself; not to act on power or brain but to be able to express my feelings and desires clearly and effortlessly.

Everything and its opposite

There are sayings, pieces of good advice, observations in books, in the family, or circulating on Facebook which I can make really good use of. And their very opposite as well. It's exactly like butter vs. margarine. There were years when the former was the Devil itself, while the latter saved lives. With margarine's heyday passing, new research came about with contradicting results. Eggs are considered harmful one year, then the next they're seen as vital as air. Wine is good for you even in pregnancy until I happen to read something to the contrary. Well, what if I don't like wine? How is that possible?! Because my body is like nobody else's. My body doesn't like wine and in many cases my soul longs for something different to millions of other people, no matter what the research says. Is the best thing to breastfeed hourly? Or should I give the baby milk every time she asks for it? Or should I feed her every four hours? Just because that's what I read somewhere, I should do neither! Feeling what's best for us both, that'll be just right. I'm the best researcher of my own life, my own body, my own child. If I like using outside affirmations as crutches, I can change the order: first find what my inner voice says and then look for the bit of wisdom or wise people who are in support of that.

My boundaries

My boundaries limit me; the way a black hole frames my space, they curtail my freedom. I can only move around in the space I can secure for myself.

When we have enough money to eat out, but I feel that sitting calmly in a restaurant with all the kids presents more difficulty than it's worth, then I actually keep myself in the habit of cooking daily.

If I feel that it's harder to go on holiday with this number of kids than to stay at home within the safety created by our routines, then I erect a barrier around me.

If I long for three days on my own and I have the chance to take them, but I don't, that also highlights my limits.

I often consider my limits tight, but still I don't label myself as limited; that's a very negative and judgemental adjective. My boundaries are not bad. They may show my value system: even though I'd like to be alone, it's still not worth it for me to take the chance. As much as I'd definitely feel recharged by it, it could take too long to heal the wound the separation would leave on the soul of my one-year-old. Boundaries can also show self-awareness: I won't go to a restaurant even though it would be better not to have to cook, but still, knowing me, I'd have to invest much more energy into getting the kids to sit peacefully at the table.

Boundaries can also show a combination of both: there are thousands of different types of holidays I could take, but I'm still at the stage when having a babysitter there with my children is not something I dream of. And to move one step back… my idea of relaxing includes the children being there. I'm fully aware that it's possible to have a holiday with just the two of us, or the three of us, with a babysitter or grandma.

My limits are boundaries that are not set in concrete. Perhaps my inner fences will move by metres tomorrow, which primarily depends on whether I dedicate enough time and energy to discover why I work the way I do. If I can't figure it out, it's up to me whether I can ask for help, whether I decide to set off to explore myself. If I manage to get closer to the roots of my mechanisms, my limits become a little more relaxed and I can instantly decide more freely about whether I want to carry on working the same way the following day as well.

Floodgates

I'm driving like crazy, stepping hard on the gas. Finally, I'll see them, I've missed them, I'm running up the stairs, I fall through the door, they're happy, telling stories, asking questions – then within five minutes we tense up and argue. This happens regularly. Why? Because I'm not yet able to be fully present for them in spirit, no matter how much I'd like to be. Part of me was longing to be with them, but the other part is still at work, with a friend, or wherever else. My intention is good, but I don't notice that I'm not doing good for them. What's the solution? Floodgates.

I sit in the car for five more minutes. I retune. I think about where I was and anticipate what I'm going into. I stop in front of the house and wait for three minutes before I walk in the door. I listen to the noises, I take deep breaths. I sense whether I've really arrived. If I haven't arrived yet but I must enter the flat because, for instance, I have to change places with the babysitter, I can actually tell the kids that I need three more minutes to go for a pee, have a shower, have a cup of tea, please. As they must have been looking forward to seeing me, it helps them if I add that afterwards I'll be all theirs, fully available for board games, conversations, and hugs.

Symbiotic

Through my child I sometimes find it much easier to experience negative emotions such as pain, anger, or shame. If the teacher is unfair to him, that can make me angrier than if it happened to me. I also feel ashamed when he farts on a crowded bus and we are angry together with the downstairs neighbour who insulted him. My symbiosis with him provides an opportunity to experience feelings together, which makes our connection stronger. However, when he has a greater, lasting, or recurrent problem and I stay in this symbiosis for too long, then we easily reach the phase of wallowing in warm manure together, whereby being in symbiosis I'm helping neither him nor myself to move on. When I sense that he could perhaps do with some help, but being at the same place I'm unable to pull or push, what can I do? I come out of the symbiotic state by putting myself somewhere else. I examine, think over, try to get an alternative view of things. If I don't succeed, I ask for the eyes of an expert, a more distant family member or a friend. I describe to them the situation, doing my best to present only the dry facts, removing my feelings and my concepts. Then I listen to what they see. The main thing is not that I accept the advice, much more that I get to see myself through somebody else's eyes in the given situation, to find layers I haven't noticed before. If I manage to distance myself from my child a little, it's highly likely that he'll also be able to move beyond the deadlock.

Touch saturation

I have a friend who puts her hand around the waist of everyone who sits down next to her for a chat. It's taken me a few years to be able to tell her not to do it to me, please. I'm not the other extreme either. I don't break out in a sweat when I'm kissed by family members on my birthday. I'm probably average in terms of my need for giving and receiving touch.

However, there is a touch saturation point which I sometimes fight, especially when I reach it with my children. As a rule, we're quite touchy-feely. There are kisses and hugs, tickles. There's a mutually agreed average daily dose of give and take. My need for touch depends on my emotional state. If I'm not well emotionally or physically, my tolerance and need for touch drops dramatically. I don't like to be touched while I'm eating. When I'm breastfeeding and there comes the second, and the third, and the fourth child to cuddle up as well, as outrageous as it is, I must admit with some unease that I've felt like pushing them away on several occasions. Even the sensation that I have no desire for any more closeness fills me with shame, that's why it's so hard to say it. And it's extremely hard to accept that the very thing that at other times is the highlight of my day can be too much for me.

My labels

Throughout my life, I've always claimed that I hate doing sports and I don't even run for the bus. I considered myself a lazy person through and through. I remember how much I hated going on excursions or walking as a child and I never understood how people could enjoy doing sports. Of course, when I think about it, I used to love riding my bike with my dad on Witches' Island in Szeged, my home town, and I loved walking my dog with my friends – it was the highlight of my days for many years. Walking the dog? Brilliant! When exercise was a joy, my legs were not made of lead. If I overcome my shyness, I love dancing as well. Still, it was as firm as a rock in my head that I hated doing sports. I found it funny, attention-drawing, special; it became a part of my identity, my creed.

Simultaneously, I was fighting with the kilos and even when I didn't have any extra weight, I was busy trying to believe that I did. The constant dieting, the dissatisfaction with myself, and the fight also defined me, became a part of me. These two things cemented me into something I was seemingly trying to break out of, but only managed to do so momentarily. I tried to break out with diets. I lost weight for a few months, but nothing changed in my mind. I still felt fat – as if the mirror was in a phase delay at those times. I tried to do sports, this and that, but just like a nerve trapped from bad posture, a few days after massaging it out, I snapped back into my "normal" state. And mostly only my mouth kept moving, not my feet. I hated myself, I was angry with myself about this and so I created permanent inner tension.

One of my friends suggested that I not think of sports as "sports", but simply as exercise. At that point something switched over. I could remain the girl who hates doing sports but just does some exercise two-three-four times a week. That's great! Since then I've been exercising regularly. It wasn't easy to find room for it in between the thousands of daily duties and activities. My children have not grown up and flown the nest from Monday to Tuesday. And, most of all, my motivation to exercise has not increased either. I just simply got fed up with saying the same things forever, and this finally resulted in a shift in me which also reached down to my feet.

However, I still don't say that I do sports – my mind leaves behind its own limits with even more difficulty than my body. I wonder in how many areas I limit myself simply by my labels.

Living up to expectations

As soon as I try to live up to anybody's expectations, when I do something differently to what would truly come from my heart, when I slide from where I feel good, disharmony is created in me. This can push me and thus anything around me further – such is the nature of the domino effect.

Is there anyone in the world who willingly gives up sleeping five-six-eight hours in one go for years? Is there a single adult in the world who sings Itsy Bitsy Spider and counts ten fingers with a rhyme regularly in weekly gatherings just for fun? Is there anybody who voluntarily and happily goes to the playground once or twice a day? Is there a living soul who mushes peas and pumpkin with breastmilk of their own accord for themselves?

It is one of the hardest things for me to rank my needs and desires before my children's, even if I know that in the long run this will serve them well, too. On the other hand, though, I wouldn't like to become a victim of raising my children. So how do I avoid that?

For example, by seeing the long and the short term at the same time. In the short term, there are many parenting tasks I don't really like doing, if I just look at the activities themselves. I would be bored to tears by the weekly music workshop if I didn't see the joy on my daughter's face, if there wasn't such a great connection between us there which makes it all worthwhile. Sometimes it's hard work and boring and a burden to figure out what to cook for the day, and keep the children busy at the same time, but then it's good to watch as they happily scoff it all down – so it's worth it. Not because of them but because it feels good to me; I like to give.

If I'm able to switch things that I don't necessarily do with joy, if I can see that I'm doing them for myself, then I can't be a victim. I decided to have the children for me, because I enjoy being with them. I enjoy witnessing as the enormous amounts of time, working, not sleeping, mashing up food, taking nightshifts, carrying-till-my-back-hurts, reducing fever, studying together, and all the other stuff bear fruit. To some extent I'm actually really selfish as, for instance, the main reason I breastfeed my child at night is so that he can grow into a securely attached, balanced bigger person, which is of great benefit to me as I get to live with a well-functioning minor and then I get to see him working well as an adult, too.

And then I have the chance to weigh things up every minute: if something really doesn't feel good and is not worth doing even for the moment of joy it offers and I am not interested in the long term either, then I just don't do it and that's that. And sometimes it happens that I really want to live up to somebody's expectations (somebody else's or my own ideals) and so I do it even though I don't really feel like doing it, and in the end, this can still feel quite good somehow. A world of a thousand colours.

Weighing up

Every day I place things on the scales and decide which way to go on. The scales used for weighing in order to make my decisions cannot be switched off; perhaps I just feel the weight on the left and right and don't check the balance.

Let's take breastfeeding, for example. On the one hand it feels terrific that I can cuddle up with a soft small body and sense his snuffling. It's important that I can give him food and security, it's great that I can bring him calm in this relatively simple way. Simultaneously, though, in the other pan of my scales, breastfeeding is not that simple at all. And here I don't only mean the technical aspects, because if I have a specific problem, I can ask an expert for help. I'm mainly thinking that this is physical work for my body which often exhausts me and is quite a strain. It's not necessarily easy to give of myself, let's say, many times a day, over two years, at the playground or when I'd rather feed myself. Even if I'm able and willing to say no to his needs in certain situations, it's not necessarily easy for me to make such decisions. Because I weigh up every single time whether to give him breastmilk or not. I weigh up whether it's easier for me to get up several times during the night to breastfeed him, or whether it would be easier for me to make some infant formula for him. And I also weigh up every time whether I'd like to carry on breastfeeding my child or wean him off. Such a lot of weighing up to do.

And sometimes my inner scales do not measure on their own. I let the health visitor lean on one of the pans and, let's say, my mother-in-law on the other; they fight in my head like gladiators in an arena. But I'm the one who puts the stuff to be measured on my scales, and I'm the one who reads the balance and makes the decisions a thousand times a day. I can see this as a burden or as thousands of small opportunities to progress towards my desired life – this is also a question of weighing up and then deciding.

It's never too late

If I get stuck in the time when my child was in my belly, and how it was yesterday, or last week, or that I didn't do this or that perfectly for years, then I miss out on the present. Did I shout at him yesterday? Ok, I feel bad about it. I can dig a hole in the ground and bury myself in it, that's all right. Then I get up, back to the surface and carry on. Let's make use of it, learn from it. Because this morning is here, and we can say sorry, I love you. I'll try to get more sleep to avoid pushing the tension built up from lack of sleep onto him. Not having breastfed for long enough or for too long or not at all? How long have I been mulling over this? Fourteen and a half years? And has it got better, has it helped me find a way to him or myself? If so, then OK. If not, then it should be seen under a different light or got rid of. Do I carry on wearing a dress for fourteen and a half years if it's not comfortable? On the one hand it's never too late to throw away my much-cherished knick-knacks; on the other it's possible to replace them with something else I can cherish – for example, my fourteen-and-a-half-year-old adolescent child.

She comes to our bed at night

I hate it. We try everything. We walk her back into her bed. I tell her in the morning that this is not good for me and could she please sleep in her own bed. Talking to her, I'm trying to discover the reason for her night visits/waking up together with her. The following day I take the crickets in the bathroom (bearded dragon food can be very noisy at night) in case that's what's waking her. We put her into bed earlier. We put her into bed later. We cover her at night in case she's feeling cold. We uncover her in case she's feeling too warm. We ask her to sleep next to one of her brothers – there are enthusiastic volunteers. Nothing works. So, unfortunately, I'll have to find some solution inside – even though it would have been so much easier to blame the crickets.

Why does it bother me, why do I feel so tense, why do I want her so desperately to sleep in her own bed? First, there is not actually enough room left for us. Her brother has a valid ticket to our bed as he's still on the breast at night and I don't want to spend half the night in an armchair. But with four of us in the bed, there's about a fifty-centimeter-wide bed space available to each of us – though the minors often manage to occupy eighty centimeters for themselves and we easily squeeze into the twenty centimeters left for us, as we have a good sixteen hours a day to get rid of our lower back pain. Second, I like to cuddle up to my husband at night; by then I've had more than enough of the children's touch and closeness. And third, there's also the fear that we won't be able to get her used to her own bed again and I don't want her to still be coming in with us in five years' time.

Perhaps I could even resign myself to her sleeping with us if these three things were not in play. The first two problems are solved by putting a small mattress at the end of the bed and telling her that's where she should sleep when she comes to our room. As for my worries about the future – I can put a stop to these rationally: I've got enough to worry about in the present without making predictions about what might happen in five years' time and how I may feel about it then. Why should I worry now about the possible solutions for then? I'll cross that bridge when I come to it. Or it may even be that it doesn't worry me at all then; I will simply look for and find a solution – just like I've done this time.

It's not fair

Why does it bother me so much that I have to sit next to my child while she falls asleep? It irritates me. It's as if a thousand ants were running around on me. With my first three children it was bedtime at 7.30 for many years. I was proud of that, I thought that it was achieved with my hard and consistent parenting, because I was such a brilliant and superb mother. Well, then, there is this fourth child here who still doesn't want to sleep at 9.30. It must be the big brothers, it must be too noisy, her bed must be in the wrong place. I ask a lactation consultant for advice about what could be done differently, and she says that there are simply children who go to bed earlier and ones who go to bed later and I won't really be able to reset this, it's biology. So that's why it has been bothering me so much! Because this actually means that so far I've just been lucky, and none of it was a triumph of my super-consistency.

Scapegoat

When they come with "He started it," I often convince them to take a look at whether they have (also) had a part in creating the situation. Not because we're looking for a scapegoat – in truth what interests me the least in an argument is who started it. I'd just like peace and quiet, not a guilty party. If I think of things happening to me as things I can shape myself and I don't place responsibility on the outside, then I can detect more effectively how I can avoid similar, unpleasant situations. Sometimes events totally removed from the given situation also play a part: for example, an earlier, unresolved grievance, or even my discomfort from feeling hungry may be enough for an explosion.

One day, my ten-year-old son came home from school saying that he had been given a grade, but it was the teacher's fault. I started my usual recording of "You know when you feel that something is somebody else's fault, it's worth considering that..." when he interrupted me and told me that the grade he'd been given was an 'A' star, and it was the teacher's fault as he had failed to spot his mistake. There goes the point.

Irritation game

He has known for two months that he has to read a book of 149 pages, but he leaves fifty pages for the night before the deadline. As soon as this comes out, I start pushing him: "If you stay awake a little longer, you can still finish it, go on, read!" Then I realise that this is a point which is just as much about me as it is about him, so I opt for the path of a half-minute introspection to see what's happening in me. The following feelings come up: feeling wedged in, feeling helpless, feeling anger due to helplessness, feeling shame and a strong sense of irritation.

When I notice that something really bothers me about my

children, it must be about me and not them. They are only indicators, bits of litmus paper. The things hidden behind my irritation are those that are often my most painful and least scratchable spots. Either irritation or a feeling of opposition erupting from the stomach with such elemental strength that it throws me away from the thing I could see and face, were I able to get close to it. However, if I'm not ready or open to facing the block, then I can throw a good dose of judgement on the matter so that it's bad/outrageous/disgusting as it is. So, if I'd like to play this self-knowledge game, I just take a few things that irritate me in my children and take a closer look at them in a way that I internalise them and taste them as part of my own character.

It irritates me that my son, for example, leaves things to the last minute and is not hard-working enough. What are the feelings that well up in me when I think that I am not hard-working enough? The first one is shame. I see myself as a small child at the school desk, in turtle pose (pulling my head down between my shoulders), eyes looking down. I'm not good enough, I haven't lived up to the teacher's expectations, I'm scorned for it, given a punishment or suffer a withdrawal of affection. Who would want that? Not me. So, I use my brain to help myself right away: it's time to grow up. I'm loveable even if I'm not hard-working, not perfect, if my homework is not always ready, if I don't prepare for a test.

Why don't you go and play football? Or a board game? Do you feel like cooking something? Have you given the animals something to eat yet? I feel irritated when they are bored. I know in my mind, as I've learnt and read about it, that being bored is the gateway to creativity: you should definitely let a child feel bored. Despite being aware of these facts, I still feel irritated when my child is not engaged in some sort of activity.

It's likely that I will find the answer or the solution somewhere inside me if I want to make a change. For a moment, I'm a bored child and I can instantly feel the lack of acceptance, and the feeling that I irritate those around me. It's not certain that this was the case every single time, but I recall that it happened several times. It comes straight up that I don't allow myself to be bored in the present either. I keep myself busy. It's far more common that I'm doing two or three things at the same time than none at all. Is it because if I do nothing then I'm good for nothing?

In fairytales, this type of association is ever so common, and those fairytales also serve as pattern providers. The young man lying on the meadow, bathing in the sun, or looking up at the starry sky for hours, not working and not contributing to the wealth of the family, well, he's a good-for-nothing fellow. I attached negative feelings to boredom as a child and as an adult these have remained the basis of my work. I'd like to change this. I'll try to be bored for ten to fifteen minutes at a time from now on and I curiously wait to see how I get on. If I succeed in recolouring the experience, I'm certain that the conflicts in this area will become fewer at home. I'll not create tension by offering ways of keeping busy to my child who's sitting on the settee, staring into space, when he doesn't feel like doing anything.

Waiting for solutions: a waste of time and energy

If I feel that I've had too much of them, I move away. When I feel they're too loud, I can close the door or turn some music on. If it's too much for me to give him dinner twice, he can make the second one for himself if he's that hungry. If it's too tiring for me to give him a drink twice a night, I can put some drink in a no-spill cup next to his bed and teach him how to drink from it. If sibling fights irritate me, I can ask my mother or mother-in-law to come over and I can go out for a walk or shut the bathroom door or hang out the washing. If I feel he's too remote, I can also try to get closer. If he is too withdrawn, I should open up to him. If I feel he spends too little time with me, I can think of something we can happily do together. If my child does not work the way I'd like him to, it's much faster and more effective for me to make a change than to wait for him to do so.

Everyone has the right to be unhappy

When my mother keeps offering me some stuff made from unidentifiable ingredients with what seems to me a repulsive texture, she calls it food and she keeps offering it to me: "Try it, it's really tasty," I find it easy to explain that there is no such thing as tasty. There's only I like it, or you like it and it's not beside the point whether I'm hungry at all in the first place. No one can tell me what tasty or beautiful is, what happiness is or what the right way is.

What do I do then? I'd like those I love to be so happy that I fail to notice at times how forcefully I push to convince them of the rightness of what I consider the way to happiness. Sometimes I have to repeat a mantra to myself saying "He has the right to be unhappy, he is entitled to be unhappy." And at the same time, it's easily possible that what I consider unhappiness is Nirvana itself to him.

Crossroads

The other day, I was really angry with my husband for spending as long as half an hour in the bathroom while I was struggling with our sick child. He was taking his time getting ready and then was off to work. I had to stay in and cope relentlessly with endless tasks. It's really great that I have some ready-to-use techniques. I could see that there was a good chance I'd jump down his throat like a rabid dog as soon as he came out of the bathroom, but I could also feel that that was not really what I wanted to do. I didn't want to fight. I didn't feel it was justified, as the problem was not what he was doing; the source of anxiety was in me. It irritated me because I couldn't do the same. There was no outside reason why I couldn't if I wanted to – I could also spend that long in the bathroom. I simply tend not to give myself permission to tear myself away from the sick child for half an hour in the morning rush. Detecting this, I managed to shift my own boundaries and instead of angry screaming or more tension I was able to tell my husband that I was ready to blow, and I didn't think it wise to be around me at the moment as there was a good chance he would be used as a punching bag. As soon as I said that, I instantly felt two kilos of anger lighter. And surprise, surprise, we didn't end up having a fight.

I don't always have the strength to look for the solution within, but it's great when I do, partly because the situation itself becomes more enjoyable, and partly because I get to pat myself on the back afterwards as I know what the outcome would have been, had I been left on automatic. I can also see what happened instead. So, the warm feeling of inner freedom permeates through me and stays with me – I'm my own person when I'm able to decide which road to take.

How do I know that he's the one?

Is he the kind of man I am happy to have children with? Can he take care of us? Can I commit to him? Will I be able to put up with him for sixty years? Even the questions are all about me, not to mention the answers. In my view. There's no such thing as "the one." I believe that it's a question of whether I can still be me by his side. Can I be the person I enjoy being? Do I want to live up to his expectations? Am I like a harpy with him, arguing all the time? Would I like him to change in many ways? Can I give myself boundlessly? Can I be myself with him? Are most days spent together days I'd be happy to relive for sixty years or not? When I'm not working the way I'd like to when I'm with him, do I feel the strength, do I have the time and the patience to find the places for change in myself? Because unfortunately or fortunately, I cannot mould him. My only chance is to change myself, to make a shift in myself, which, of course, may cause shifts in our relationship and result in a domino effect, too.

Board game

Together and supporting one another. These are the two things that provide the basis for me to be able to perform to the best of my ability as a mother. When I have a partner with whom I can shape the circles of our parental responsibilities without hierarchy – he tidies up and I make lunch; he works, I breastfeed; I work, he takes the children to the playground – then I work well as a mother. If he supports me with his actions in being the mother I want to be according to my own value system, daily life rolls on. If I support him in taking part in parenting according to his own needs, to work if he chooses to or to stay at home on paternity leave if he wishes to do so, he'll work well, too. By supporting and helping him to become a competent, fully functioning father, I'm not only giving him the chance to enjoy being a parent, but I'm also giving a lot to myself. He'll not be second to me, but he'll be just as important to and responsible for the children as me. If we can weave together our needs and desires, if both our individual and our common goals are of the utmost importance, there aren't really any insurmountable problems.

There isn't a single day that we don't both have to work on this. In the first round, we need to communicate continuously about what's happening inside, what has changed since the previous day, what we want in the long and short term. Everything from putting the children to bed in half an hour to whether I'd like to return to work the following spring. In order to keep communicating, monitoring myself day by day or even a number of times a day is essential: am I living the life I'd like to live? Is our daily life something I can be happy with? Is my life taking me closer to my long-term desires? It takes an awful lot of energy to listen inwardly and outwardly and express even those things that are unimaginable as yet or knock on taboos. It takes courage to assert myself when I think that my partner wouldn't agree with me or when my desires clash with his. Sometimes I have to conquer shame and fear in order to do that. Still, it's important to do so because open and honest communication is a great tool for happiness. My partner can see my needs and I know of his, so we can start thinking of solutions separately and together. If there's constant feedback, we detect distancing and thus we have the opportunity to find a way back to each other, so there's less chance of discovering unexpectedly that we've grown apart over the years.

Career vs. children

Children=self-surrender? Is it the end of my career? Do my work achievements and recognition dissolve into thin air? Is it possible to stay the same person?

When I think back to why I wanted children in the first place, the first thing I can think of is for it to change my life. If the soup tastes great the way it is, do I carry on adding more spices? When I say let that baby come, I also say, let it change things, bring new colour!

The way I relate to change depends on me and not on change itself. I can take it as an experience: I see it as a challenge that I long to discover. Or I can relate to it with fear. I can dread losing the old things, fretting that the new may present unfavourable layers to my life. Of course, a mixture of all these is the most common reaction to change. The more extreme and permanent I see change, the scarier it looks.

Can I remain the person I've been so far? If I identify with my work or my daily routine, for instance I'm the best hairdresser in the district, or I'm a person who reads the paper with her coffee every morning, then my identity will be deeply affected by change. Having a child will be frightening; it'll seem as if I am losing myself as well by doing something different.

If I collect my daily drops of happiness in my workplace, in the form of words of appreciation, utterances of approval, or a salary, then I'll find it hard to switch. Who would want to lose their titbits of reward? I'll definitely find these in my new life situation, but it's hard to imagine where until I'm actually living my new life.

Choosing mothering over my job can also be scary because I know my job while I don't know how to be with my child yet. I know myself as a working person, but I haven't met my mother-me yet. If I can only hold onto things in my head, the change is frightening. Before the conception of my first child, I don't have any knowledge about what's good in all of this for me on the level of feelings and actions. It's like moving to a new country: my house will be different, there'll also be different people around me. I'll have to learn a new language. I'll have to do well in an unknown situation. Many new things will happen to me and yes, there'll be certain things I'll really miss from my old life. There'll also be many things I won't miss at all if I really long for change.

My old life, my work, may be pursued in my new country as well, even if not in an unaltered form. It's possible to stay at home for three years, put the baby in a nursery after six months, leave him at home with a grandmother, a grandfather, a babysitter, and so on. There are many ways of doing things and I don't necessarily need to make a decision about these before conception or before having a child. It helps dissolve the blocks in me when I think that I have the time and space to think over my decisions.

Just because I've had children, I'm still the same person, I just do different things in most parts of the day. That's because I've entered a new life phase and I'd like to do different things. However, I can also do what I used to do again; the form it takes is a question of my motivation and my decision.

If I examine and recognise my own desires and I also have the courage to fight for them, then I can trust myself; maybe not right away but with perseverance I'll be able to find the work-life balance that suits everyone.

When is it ideal to have a baby?

Am I longing for a child? Am I longing for my life to change? Yes? Then, now is the time. It doesn't depend on financial wellbeing, on how old I am, on what position I have at work, on how old my previous child is, on what's recommended by parents, or on whether my friend is expecting a baby. However, I can use all of these to explore where the desire is within. Because those damn desires are really good at hiding.

There's a clear situation when I long for a child, and so does my partner. So, we decide and produce.

There's also the case when I don't really long for a child, but I force myself to want one because, for instance, my husband really longs for one, or because I'm being pressurised by many people around me. Decisions made from living up to expectations smear the process and the relationship. They can lead down paths that are hard to switch. They can have a knock-on effect, like dominoes. They can, for example, take things so far that I might experience my child or motherhood as a burden, which in turn pushes me further away as I feel guilty and try to live up to even more expectations. I get into a vicious circle and I deprive myself of the opportunity of enjoying happy everydays. However, even if my child is conceived like that, it's never too late to reset my mind. Instead of bouncing around in the guilt-victim-anger triangle, I can embrace my decision and recolour it.

I long for a child, but when I conceive I'd like to back out: I hate the whole idea, I'd rather have an abortion. I may fear pregnancy, birth, or commitment so much that I stop feeling desire and just want to run away. Just like when I'm flooded with fear, I run away instinctively, or I freeze. If I can find the exact source of my fear, which can be as far back as a trauma around my birth, it'll become friendlier, easier to tackle and as it gets smaller, I can feel my desire return, too.

There's also the case when I do feel desire and I don't, all at the same time. I'd like a child but equally I'd like to remain super sexy. I'd like to have a child, but I'd also like to work. I'd like to have a child, but who wants to be kept up at night all the time? It helps me not to see things in the extreme, as detached. OK, I'll be happy, but I can lose weight afterwards and it's up to me how much time and energy I put into reaching that goal. OK, the baby will probably cry and ask to be fed many times at night, but it's up to me whether I feed him or wean him off. I can even give him formula and agree with his dad to take over the night shift. Similarly, it's less extreme to say that I long for a child but I wouldn't like to try this month. I don't give up on the idea in the long term, but due to my decision I won't spend much of the given month brooding over the question.

If something is in sharp contrast with my desires or my value system, I don't have to go in that direction, but it's good to see that I could decide to do so. It's important to notice that it's not my husband, my fate, my mother-in-law, my mother, or anybody else who's responsible for whatever decision I make.

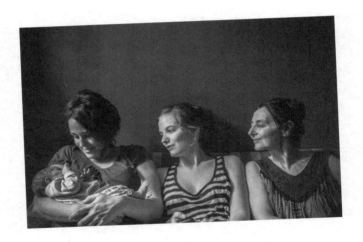

Epilogue

I started my book eighteen months ago by simply writing down what had happened the previous day. And this is the way I shall finish, too. I shall describe my yesterday.

It is the beginning of August. Schools have been out for seven weeks, and we're in the thick of summer. For the past ten days, the thermometer has been stuck at 38°C, and the heat is driving me to distraction. We're off for a holiday, two weeks at Lake Balaton. Packing has never been my favourite task. The two under-fours ask me every single minute when we're leaving. The adolescents sit on the settee, dreamy-eyed and as motionless as chameleons, with their empty rucksacks gaping open-mouthed at them. The pre-pubescent child is all packed. He's interested in what we're going to have for lunch. My husband and I are running around, clocking up miles in the apartment to assemble our thoughts and collect items we might still need on our holiday. Exhausted and relatively conflict-free, we finally reach the "Is everyone strapped in?" moment. The house that we are renting is tiny, a third of our living space at home. Never mind, it's only an-hour-and-a-half journey and we can all bathe and relax in the long-deserved waters. But a blast of wind and a scattering of hailstones beats us to it by about twenty minutes. We are stuck. In the house and in ourselves. The big boys are killing each other; first blood has been drawn. The little ones take it in turns to cry. A snail proceeds backwards faster than time crawls forwards, towards the oh-so-desired bedtime. I'm in the worst state. For a long time, I successfully navigate my own and everybody else's tension in different ways, but towards the end of the day I finally explode. My impatience, my anger, my irritation erupt, and I start to shout and curse, though I don't usually swear. A passing witness might fairly ask: so, is this the mother who is writing a book about raising children?

What I read in my previous paragraph is uplifting. I'm relieved that I can honestly depict a side of myself which is also me. I don't feel crushed by shame. I don't hide. I can turn myself inside out. I'm not very proud of what I lay bare, but I am proud of the fact that I don't only see the bad in it all. I also notice that there's been nothing like this in the past five or six months, even though years ago we reached similar depths at least once a week, for sure. I'm proud of not hating myself, of accepting that there are rubbish days. I don't drown in a cycle of guilt, I don't do penance, I don't beg for forgiveness. I've known for a while that these never take me forward, but I tend to work instinctively along these lines more and more often. I examine what I'd do differently on other occasions, in order to less frequently get into the state I was in yesterday. I'd like to make myself prettier inside, and it's good that there is still stuff to do.

I still had plenty left over from yesterday's tension, so I decided not to label the sweeping energy inside me but use it instead and go running. And now that movement has resolved that tension inside me, I can write again. I can write an ending to my book after what has been a good year.

P.S. It makes no difference what's going on inside me; the question is what I do with it. My motivation for writing this book was to pay my sons' school fees. My publisher warned me at our very first meeting that my plan was mistaken. By the time I got to the publishers, I realised that this lack of money and my desire to break out of this situation served as an excellent springboard, a great incentive to start moving toward myself. Had circumstances not squeezed me this way, I suspect I'd have postponed my search at least until my one-year-old went to kindergarten. I might have let my desires hibernate for years. People ask me how and when I could write a book with five children around. My question is how I could have managed to get through the past year without writing. Three or four times a week the world was mine between 5 and 7.30 in the morning. I got some me-time, time to recharge, space to look inwards, silence.

After finishing the book, I kept the early hours for myself, to exercise and be alone with my thoughts. I know for sure that I'd have been less able to be emotionally accessible to my children over the past eighteen months if I hadn't changed a thing. I was so totally saturated by years spent being with children and missing the freedom of adulthood so much, that the outside pressure came at the best possible time. I assume that as a good industrious mother I'd have got through this period with a grade of C or a B-. I'd often have been emotionally unavailable for my children, for example, which could have caused them as much separation anxiety as spending most of the day apart. The goal I have reached, my book, and what it shows by coming into existence, is that I recognise where I can shape my life, and thus my children's, to find even greater happiness. I do a lot for it, which is a great liberty and a treasure. Whether my book brings material wealth is immaterial; I am rich already.

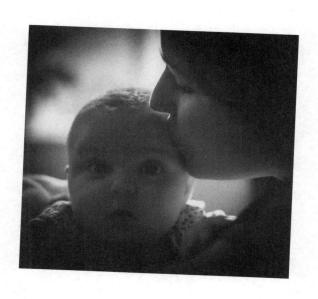